# PAIN—New Perspectives in Measurement and Management

# PAIN—New Perspectives in Measurement and Management

EDITED BY

A. W. HARCUS, M.B.Ch.B., D.Obst.R.C.O.G.
*Head of Medical Affairs*
*Pharmaceutical Division, Reckitt & Colman*

R. B. SMITH, B.Sc., M.B.Ch.B., M.D., Dip.Pharm. Med.
*International Development and Medical Director*
*Pharmaceutical Division, Reckitt & Colman*

B. A. WHITTLE, B.Pharm., F.P.S., M.Sc., Ph.D.
*Head of Regulatory Affairs*
*Pharmaceutical Division, Reckitt & Colman*

FOREWORD BY

Professor G. V. R. Born, F.R.C.P., F.R.S.
*Shield Professor of Pharmacology*
*University of Cambridge*

CHURCHILL LIVINGSTONE
EDINBURGH LONDON AND NEW YORK 1977

CHURCHILL LIVINGSTONE
Medical Division of Longman Group Limited

Distributed in the United States of America by
Longman Inc., 19 West 44th Street, New York,
N.Y. 10036 and by associated companies,
branches and representatives throughout
the world.

ISBN   0  443   01745  X

British Library Cataloguing in Publication Data
Pain.
   1. Pain - Congresses
   I. Harcus, A W   II. Smith, R B
   III. Whittle, B A
   616'.047        RB127        77-30592

Printed in Great Britain by Lowe & Brydone, Thetford, England.

# Foreword

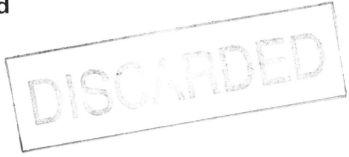

This symposium on pain and its relief by drugs comes at an opportune time because the last few years have seen the most important discoveries in analgesic pharmacology since that of the volatile anaesthetics more than a hundred years ago. One of these discoveries is the mode of the analgesic action of aspirin through the inhibition of prostaglandin biosynthesis (Vane, 1971; Fereira, 1972); and another is the demonstration of brain peptides with analgesic actions similar to morphine (Hughes, Smith, Kosterlitz, Fothergill, Morgan & Morris, 1975). As a result, hypotheses about pain mechanisms and their inhibition have at last received a scientific basis, and it is now realistic to expect this rapidly increasing understanding to bring about improvements in clinical management.

The first part of this book is devoted to psychological, physiological and pharmacological aspects of pain. As pain shows itself primarily psychologically, its quantification has always been difficult. Therefore, the two chapters dealing with measurement of pain are particularly valuable. Furthermore, it is highly appropriate that the chapter on pharmacological advances in analgesia should be by Professor H.W. Kosterlitz, whose classical contributions to knowledge about the agonist/antagonist properties of the opiate analgesics were made by measurements with the simple guinea-pig ileum preparation and whose imaginative awareness made him a co-discoverer of the analgesic peptides.

The latter part of the book provides good accounts of the strong analgesic buprenorphine, which has recently been introduced into clinical practice. This drug was developed from the morphine analogues discovered by Professor K.W. Bentley (Bentley, Hardy & Meek, 1967; Bentley & Hardy, 1967), the analgesic potency of which is several orders of magnitude greater than that of morphine itself. This drug has a distribution of opiate properties which appear to give it singular advantages in a number of clinically common situations. That this is so shows that real advances in modern analgesia remain possible on the basis of a drug effect that has been known for thousands of years.

Prof. G.V.R. Born, F.R.C.P., F.R.S.
Shield Professor of Pharmacology,
University of Cambridge

## References

Bentley, K.W., Hardy, D.G. & Meek, B. (1967). *J. Amer. Chem. Soc.,* **89**, 3273 − 3280.
Bentley, K.W. & Hardy, D.G. (1976). *J. Amer. Chem. Soc.,* **89**, 3281 − 3292.
Fereira, S.H. (1972). *Nature New Biology,* **240**, 200 − 203.
Hughes, J., Smith, T.W., Kosterlitz, H.W., Fothergill, L.A., Morgan, B.A. & Morris, H.R. (1975).
*Nature, Lond.,* **258**, 577 − 579.
Vane, J.R. (1971). *Nature New Biology,* **231**, 232 − 235.

# Preface

Pain concerns us all and is probably the most common reason why patients seek the help of a physician. The existence of pain has been a constant stimulus to the discovery of both substances and procedures for the relief of pain.

Naturally occurring agents such as opium were known in antiquity, but it was not until the early years of the nineteenth century that the active principles of these anodynes were isolated, characterised and later synthesised. The search for more effective and safer analgesics, by the pharmaceutical industry and clinical trialists, has not only provided the physician with improved agents but has, in the process, also refined the methodology of pharmaceutical and clinical research into pain. It is significant that the most potent synthetic analgesics are still derived from opium, and their development has been made possible only by unravelling some of the secrets of these older compounds. The most recent discovery of substances in the brain which have analgesic characteristics opens up a fascinating vista.

This book is based on a two-day symposium held in May 1977. The symposium brought together physicians, surgeons and scientists from academic and research institutes, clinical practice and the pharmaceutical industry. It provided a forum for the exchange of specialist views on many aspects of the management of pain. The words of Peter Mere Latham (1789—1875) are still an accurate summary of the state of the art and express our thoughts in arranging this symposium:-

'It would be a great thing to understand pain in all its meanings'.

We wish to thank our distinguished Chairmen and participants for their ready co-operation, the States of Guernsey for their help and hospitality and the publishers, Churchill Livingstone, for their collaboration.

We are especially grateful to Miss H. Taylor for preparation of the tables, Miss S. Townend and her colleagues in the Medical Department of the Pharmaceutical Division of Reckitt & Colman for preparation of the manuscripts. We also thank Mr E.F. Engler for his help with the references, and Mr. A.R. Tettenborn for his help with the proof reading.

A.W.H., R.B.S., B.A.W.

# Authors and participants

J.I. Alexander, M.B., B.S., M.R.C.S., L.R.C.P., F.F.A.R.C.S., D.Obst. R.C.O.G.
*Consultant Anaesthetist, Bristol Royal Infirmary.*

J. Bertram, F.R.C.S., M.Ch. (Orth).
*Consultant in Orthopaedics, Royal Naval Hospital, Plymouth.*

P.L.T. Bevan, B.Sc., Ph.D.
*Senior Medical Sciences Executive (International), Reckitt & Colman, Hull.*

T.H. Bewley, M.A., M.D., F.R.C.P.I., F.R.C.Psych.
*Consultant Psychiatrist, St Thomas' and Tooting Bec Hospital, London.*

F.B. Buckley, B.Sc., Ph.D., F.I. Biol.
*Medical Department, Reckitt & Colman, Hull.*

K. Budd, M.B., Ch.B., F.F.A.R.C.S.
*Consultant Anaesthetist, Bradford Royal Infirmary.*

J.M.B. Burn, M.B., Ch.B., F.F.A.R.C.S., D.Obst. R.C.O.G.
*Consultant Anaesthetist, Southampton General Hospital.*

D. Campbell, M.B., Ch.B., F.F.A.R.C.S., D.A.
*Professor of Anaesthesia, University of Glasgow.*

M.D. Churcher, M.B., B.S., F.F.A.R.C.S.
*Consultant Anaesthetist, Plymouth General Hospital.*

R.S.J. Clarke, Ph.D., M.D., F.F.A.R.C.S.
*Reader in Anaesthetics, The Queen's University of Belfast.*

D.J. Coltart, M.D., M.R.C.P.
*Consultant Physician, St Thomas' Hospital, London.*

M.E. Dodson, M.D., F.F.A.R.C.S.
*Senior Lecturer in Anaesthetics, University of Manchester.*

I Donald, C.B.E., B.A., M.D., F.R.C.S. (Glas.), F.R.C.O.G., F.C.O.G. (S.A), F.A.C.O.G.
*Emeritus Professor of Midwifery, University of Glasgow.*

J.W. Dundee, Ph.D., M.D., M.R.C.P. (Lon.), F.F.A.R.C.S.(I), F.F.A.R.C.S. (Eng.), B.A.
*Professor of Anaesthetics, The Queen's University of Belfast.*

P. Edmond, F.R.C.S. (Ed.)
*Consultant Surgeon, The Royal Infirmary, Edinburgh.*

M. Footerman, M.R.C.S. (Lon.), L.R.C.P. (Lon.)
*Guernsey.*

E.N.S. Fry, M.B., Ch.B., F.F.A.R.C.S., D.A. (Lon.)
*Consultant Anaesthetist, North Tees General Hospital, Stockton-on-Tees.*

I.C. Geddes, M.D., F.F.A.R.C.S., D.A.
*Reader in Anaesthesia, The University of Liverpool.*

C. Glynne, M.Sc., M.B., F.F.A.R.C.S.
*Research Fellow, Abingdon Hospital, Abingdon.*

J.D.P. Graham, D.S.C., M.D., F.R.C.P., F.R.S.E., F.R.F.P.S.
*Professor of Pharmacology, University of Wales, Cardiff.*

F.R. Gusterson, B.Sc., M.B., B.S., F.F.A.R.C.S.
*Medical Director, St Barnabas Hospital, Sussex.*

J.R. Hampton, D.M., D.Phil. (Oxon)., F.R.C.P.
*Reader in Medicine, University of Nottingham.*

J.G. Hannington-Kiff, B.Sc. (Lon.), M.B., B.S., F.F.A.R.C.S.
*Consultant Anaesthetist, Frimley Park Hospital, Camberley.*

A.W. Harcus, M.B., Ch.B., D.Obst. R.C.O.G.
*Head of Medical Affairs, Reckitt & Colman, Hull.*

M.W. Hayward, B.Sc.
*Product Manager, Reckitt & Colman, Hull.*

K.E.F. Hobbs, Ch.M., F.R.C.S.
*Professor of Surgery, Royal Free Hospital School of Medicine, London.*

R.W. Houde, M.D.
*Attending Physician, Sloan Kettering Memorial Hospital, New York.*

B.C. Hovell, M.B., Ch.B., F.F.A.R.C.S.
*Consultant Anaesthetist, Hull Royal Infirmary.*

A. Hussain, M.D., F.F.A.R.C.S.
*Consultant Anaesthetist, Birch Hill Hospital, Rochdale.*

I.M. James, Ph.D., M.B., B.S., F.R.C.P.
*Senior Lecturer in Medicine and Therapeutics, The Royal Free Hospital School of Medicine, London.*

S.M. Jennett, Ph.D., M.D.
*Senior Lecturer in Physiology, University of Glasgow.*

B. Jennett, M.D., F.R.C.S. (Glas.)
*Professor of Neurosurgery, University Department of Neuro-surgery, Southern General Hospital, Glasgow.*

C.A.F. Joslin, M.I.E.R.E., C.Eng., M.B., B.S., F.R.C.R.
*Professor of Radiotherapy and Head of University Department of Radiotherapy, Leeds.*

M.M. Kamel, M.B., B.Ch., M.D., D.A., F.F.A.R.C.S.I.
*Honorary Senior Registrar, The University of Liverpool*

J.W. King, S.R.N., D.N., F.A.I.M.
*Medical Marketing Manager, Reckitt & Colman, Hull.*

H.W. Kosterlitz., M.D., Ph.D., D.Sc.,
*Director, Unit for Research on Addictive Drugs, University of Aberdeen.*

D.C. Laidlow, M.B., B.S., M.R.C.S., L.R.C.P., F.F.A.R.C.S.
*Convenor of the Intensive Care Team, Princess Elizabeth Hospital, Guernsey.*

J.W. Lewis, M.A., D.Phil.
*Scientific Director, Reckitt & Colman, Hull.*

J.W. Lloyd, M.A., F.F.A.R.C.S.
*Consultant Anaesthetist, Abingdon Hospital, Abingdon.*

K.D. MacRae, M.A., Ph.D.
*Senior Lecturer in Statistics, Charing Cross Hospital Medical School, London.*

A.D. Malcolm, M.Sc., M.B., F.R.C.P. (C)
*Senior Registrar, Cardiac Department, St Thomas' Hospital, London.*

A.H.B. Masson, F.F.A.R.C.S.
*Consultant Anaesthetist, Chalmers Hospital, Edinburgh.*

H.A.C. Matheson, M.B., Ch.B., (Glasgow), F.F.A.R.C.S.
*Senior Registrar, Manchester Royal Infirmary*

M.D. Mehta, F.F.A.R.C.S.
*Consultant Anaesthetist, Norfolk and Norwich Hospital, Norwich.*

B.V. Mooney, F.I.M.L.T.
*Pharmaceutical Manager, Reckitt's (Ireland) Ltd., Dublin.*

J.M. Orwin, M.B., Ch.B., F.F.A.R.C.S., D.A.
*Head of Clinical Pharmacology, Reckitt & Colman, Hull.*

J. Parkhouse, M.A., M.D., M.Sc., F.F.A.R.C.S.
*Professor of Anaesthetics, University of Manchester.*

E.L. Parrish,
*International Marketing Manager, Reckitt & Colman, Hull.*

D.R. Potter, M.B., B.S., F.F.A.R.C.S.
*Consultant Anaesthetist, King's College Hospital, London.*

H. Raftery, M.B., D.A., F.F.A.R.C.S.I.
*Consultant Anaesthetist, Our Lady's Hospital for Children, Dublin.*

E.G. Rees-Jones, M.D., M.B., Ch.B., D.A.
*Consultant Anaesthetist, Park Hospital, Manchester.*

D.S. Robbie, F.F.A.R.C.S.,
*Consultant Anaesthetist, The Royal Marsden Hospital, London.*

A. Rodger, B.Sc (Med. Sc.)., M.B., Ch.B., F.R.C.S. (Ed.)
*Registrar, Radiotherapy Institute, Western General Hospital, Edinburgh.*

M. Rosen, M.D., B.Ch., F.F.A.R.C.S.
*Consultant Anaesthetist, University Hospital of Wales, Cardiff.*

F.L. Rosenfeldt, M.B., B.S., M.D., F.R.C.S. (Ed.)
*Research Fellow and Lecturer in Surgery, St Thomas' Hospital, London.*

I.T. Scoular, B.Sc., Ph.D., M.I. Biol.
*Medical Department, Reckitt & Colman, Hull.*

R.B. Smith, B.Sc., M.B., Ch.B., M.D., Dip. Pharm. Med.
*International Development and Medical Director, Reckitt & Colman, Hull.*

E.I. Tate, M.B., B.S., F.F.A.R.C.S.
*Consultant Anaesthetist, Royal Victoria Infirmary, Newcastle-upon-Tyne.*

A.E. Ward, B.Sc., M.B., Ch.B.
*Medical Department, Reckitt & Colman, Hull.*

G.S. Watson, F.R.C.S. (Ed.)
*Senior Registrar, The Royal Infirmary, Edinburgh.*

W.G. Wenley, F.R.C.P.
*Consultant in Rheumatology and Rehabilitation, Norfolk and Norwich Hospital, Norwich.*

T.S. West, O.B.E., M.B., B.S.
*Deputy Medical Director, St Christopher's Hospice, London.*

B.A. Whittle, B. Pharm., F.P.S., M.Sc., Ph.D.
*Head of Regulatory Affairs, Reckitt & Colman, Hull.*

E. Wilkes, O.B.E., F.R.C.P., F.R.C.G.P., M.R.C. Psych.
*Professor of Community Care and General Practice, University of Sheffield Medical School.*

# Contents

# Session 1 Chairman: J. Parkhouse

# 1. Pain—a patient's view

IAN DONALD

Three heart operations, the last two of them on cardiopulmonary bypass, and three stays in the Intensive Care Unit have taught me quite a lot about pain in the course of the last 16 years. First of all, as a surgeon I have inflicted a good deal of pain in my life – I trust not unnecessarily. As an obstetrician I have witnessed intermittent pain, which is worse, I trust with compassion, and, I think I can say, as a patient, that I have suffered pain maximally.

Even a Resident knows that sternal marrow puncture is a very painful little operation. Multiply that by about a hundred to have some idea of a mid-sternal split. This, of course, is aggravated by essentials like breathing, and even more so by coughing, and catastrophically so by sneezing. The obstetrician, for his part, learns to observe intermittent pain, and I have always felt that it is possible for the human frame to get used to anything except pain which is intermittent such as that seen in labour at its worst.

There are many things that make pain worse, such as the spirit in which it is inflicted and I refer to the modern practices of torture which characterise our age. The spirit in which the pain is inflicted makes a great difference to a patient's acceptance or struggling against it.

From my own case and from studying others, I am in a position to make some observations which are both general and particular. Dealing with the general first: there is no doubt that the state of mind is paramount and of more importance than the most potent pain relieving drugs. As we know, the state of mind can be conditioned, first of all, by past experience and, secondly, by fear; not so much fear of death, 'that bourne from which no traveller returns', but fear, particularly in cardiovascular surgery, of a crippling neurological defect.

On both counts I was at a disadvantage: for instance, my own sister, who had similar surgery to myself, suffered an hypoxic midbrain lesion, gangrene of the toes and anuria, from all of which she ultimately died; I was 'for the chop' not much later.

It makes a difference to know that everyone is supporting you. It is also a help to know something about what you are in for, because the operation does not then come as quite such a surprise as my first heart operation, when I had not foreseen how disagreeable thoracotomy can be – far worse than laparotomy.

The absence of sympathy from attendants, whether it be in the form of silence, reticence, off-handedness or even frank apparent callousness, must make capital punishment for the criminal on his way to the gallows a particularly ugly and painful

1

experience. Dr Samuel Johnson was right when he made that brutal jest 'Depend upon it, Sir, when a man knows he is to be hanged in a fortnight, it concentrates his mind wonderfully'. You are indeed acutely vulnerable to the attitude of people surrounding you.

The importance of the preoperative personal visit by the anaesthetist the day before operation has never been stressed sufficiently. He is the first person with whom you are really going to come into contact when you face your operation. Secondly, a nurse, whom you know, accompanying you to the theatre makes a powerful difference. These two things alone are worth more than premedicating drugs.

From my practice in obstetrics, like others, I have learned the tremendous value of brain-washing in conditioning a patient's response or likely response to fear. It makes a great difference to the need or the earliness with which pain-relieving drugs are required in labour, and with adequate brain-washing, of course, labour can be made very much less painful; this is part of the business of ante-natal preparation.

However, when drugs have to be used it is better to use them before psychological decompensation sets in rather than after, when their effect is already likely to be undermined.

Of the particular observations I have to make I would like to say that the memory of pain, as we all know, fades mercifully and very quickly, but the scars which it inflicts do remain. Therefore, on the last two occasions I took the trouble to make notes as soon as I was able, and have published accounts of both these operations (Donald, 1969, 1976).

Communication with an endotracheal tube *in situ* is impossible and I was handicapped at first by the sheer inability to write because of intention tremor which is a feature of a very prolonged and hazardous anaesthetic. It took my anaesthetists quite a long time to decipher the best writing that I could contrive as the curare wore off (Fig. 1.1).

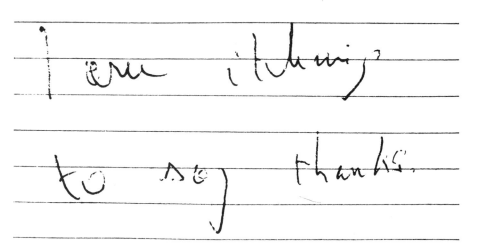

Fig. 1.1 Specimen of handwriting in the immediate post-operative period.

Pain can reach saturation point; I am sure there is no doubt of that. But it can be to some extent prevented by various methods which mitigate the intermittent horror of it. Curare and curare class drugs have an extraordinary value in this respect, which rather astonished me. I had always been brought up to fear awakening in the course of an operation, paralysed, helpless and unable to do anything for myself under the influence of a paralysing drug. In fact, the inability to struggle lessens the pain. Struggling, groaning and protesting,which make pain worse, are prevented by curare.

The endotracheal tube is a horrid thing to have and very painful in the mouth, especially if wrapped around with bandages. Pain would have prevented me from breathing properly and I was grateful to have the ventilator to do it for me. I would not have ventilated myself had it not been for the fact that I was curarised and unable to stop the ventilator. When I was seen to be registering pain I was quickly given intravenous Omnopon or some such drug.

On first regaining consciousness you are very acutely aware of intense pain, although it is difficult at first to localise. There is a certain disbelief that the operation is over. The importance of an anaesthetist telling a patient that it is 'all over' and making sure that the fact has been registered is very great. I missed out on this and I was sure it was only a half-time interval with worse to come. You wake up in unfamiliar surroundings with unfamiliar staff and your brain works extremely fast. You notice the time of day; you notice how hateful the tube is and the frustration at being unable to communicate is very real. You also notice, or at least I did, in a technical sense how scanty were my bronchial secretions when they stuck tubes down my endotracheal tube and sucked out what seemed to be a minimal quantity of mucus, thanks to having given up the filthy habit of smoking about 20 years ago.

You are not exactly grateful for drugs, but they do change the time of day or night as you surface, and you notice that it is tomorrow afternoon or the middle of the night. You do notice the time very much, and drugs pass the time quite strikingly. But in the next few days there are some very ugly, painful things to face, such as the withdrawal of tubes and drains from the pericardium and from the pleural cavity. I was astonished and unconvinced when it was suggested that this be done under a combination of entonox (nitrous oxide and oxygen mixture) and diazepam. I did not believe it would work. In fact it was remarkably effective. They said, 'we have done it', and I was not aware that the hideous job which I well remembered from previous operations was, on this occasion, totally painless. I was surprised that this combination could be so effective.

The later effects of an experience of this sort are more vividly remembered than the immediate, and of these the ones that matter particularly are the psychosomatic sequelae. The initial euphoria of having survived quickly gives way to acute depression. In obstetrics we recognise what I call 'fourth day puerperal blues'. After a major surgical operation it comes about 10 days later with nightmares, a great lack of confidence and the most irrational terrors, which I remember very acutely indeed. Quite minor things upset you — like retention of urine, or constipation induced by drugs such as Distalgesic and DF 118.

They are very upsetting matters to a patient, who suddenly attaches tremendous importance to them. Vomiting I had none of, except due to iron, which I soon refused. Recovery is made better by physiotherapy, particularly group physiotherapy, and at Hammersmith Hospital, where I was treated for the last two operations, the group physiotherapy was of a very high standard indeed.

I felt all along that you have got to be careful to deny yourself the opportunity for refusing to do anything you do not want to do, on the grounds that you have got a built-in excuse already; but that is part of the discipline of recovery.

This book is mainly about pain, not about discipline. The way pain is suffered, the way in which it is suffered by a patient, I have always felt to be more important than the actual extent of that pain itself. Pain-relieving drugs are mainly necessary when psychosomatic props, by whatsoever means, become inadequate.

The problem is how to turn anything disagreeable like this to some good account. It is for this reason that I am ready to talk or to write about it, in the hope of helping others. Whenever I go back to my old unit I am always asked to see patients who are terrified because they are about to have this kind of surgery or who feel that they will never work again, particularly doctors. There are many doctors who get treated in that unit, and once or twice I have met fellows crumpled up, refusing to put their shoulders back and saying they would never get back to work, I just bang my chest and say, 'Well, within nine weeks of both my last two operations I did my first vaginal hysterectomies as before, and I think, reasonably well'.

The idea has to be got across to people that recovery from this kind of curable condition must be absolute to make it worthwhile. Convalescence should be discouraged as far as possible, and one should encourage the patient to get back to work at once — as I did, and nobody stopped me.

The letters which I have had from doctors, from other countries and from different parts of this country, thanking me for describing my experience, have made me feel that I am right, not just to make an exhibition of myself, but to try and describe what the patient does feel about it, and what he can feel about it, given the necessary sympathetic attention which I received, and also the necessary knowledge, realising that everybody was doing their best. Above all I would hope that it has made me a better doctor.

This leads me to end up with a little rhyme, whose origin I cannot at the moment trace:

> Existence is more than the taking of breath;
> There is more to the gift than the giving.
> And dying is more than the moment of death
> And Life's more than a matter of living.

### References

Donald, I. (1969), At the receiving end; a doctor's personal recollections of valve replacement. *Lancet*, **2**, 1129-1131.

Donald, I. (1976), At the receiving end: a doctor's personal recollection of second-time valve replacement. *Scottish Medical Journal*, **21**, 49-57.

# 2. Assessment of patients with pain

R. W. HOUDE

I shall approach pain from the point of view of an internist engaged in the clinical evaluation of new putative analgesic drugs and other measures intended to relieve pain. My experience in this field has been primarily with cancer patients to whom pain and suffering are not strangers.

Although pain is a subjective matter which is uncommonly difficult to define in precise terms (Beecher, 1959) there are surely some characteristics about which I think we would all agree!As Professor Donald has so eloquently stated, pain hurts! It is a sensory experience commanding a response which, even when not expressed verbally, may be reflected in one's behaviour and often in other physical signs. It has long been known moreover, that pain has a dual nature, a cognitive and an affective component, and that sensation and reaction to pain are closely interlinked. All of these factors undoubtedly play some part in how we physicians judge the presence, severity and significance of pain in our patients. Nevertheless, in practice, as well as in our research, we rely chiefly on the patients' verbal expressions of their feelings and only perhaps to a lesser degree on their behaviour and associated physical signs.

## Patient selection

When the circumstantial factors or overt objective signs are such that we should not hesitate to ascribe them to or associate them with pain, our decisions are easily made and, quite understandably, it is this kind of patient that we seek for our studies of new drugs or other methods of relieving pain. In general, however, the decisions are not that easy to make and, when embarking on any investigation of pain or its treatment, pitfalls in the design or conduct of the study which may mislead us into attributing the outcome to the wrong thing must be carefully avoided. Part of our problem is that we are most often concerned with alleviating suffering, and the distinctions between pain and suffering may not be that clear. Pain undoubtedly causes suffering, but all suffering is not due to pain. In addition, our best efforts are frequently not rewarded by complete relief of pain in our patients and, as a rule, drugs merely serve to obtund or diminish pain, or, as many feel, to modify reaction to pain so that it is more tolerable. Thus we tend to speak of pain, and measure our success or failure in treating pain, in terms of verbal self reports of pain severity or intensity.

Although the intensity of the sensory component of pain has been generally accepted as the most salient dimension of painful experience, this premise has not gone unquestioned. A recent psychological study of Canadian university student volunteers with and without medical backgrounds addressed itself to the significance of the language of pain (Bailey, Davidson, 1976). Factor analysis of pain-descriptive adjectives revealed that intensity seemed to be distributed more in an 'affective-evaluative' than in a 'sensory' factorial space. This suggests that, as Professor Donald seems to imply, if a patient's attention can be shifted from the intensity domain to the sensory qualities of the experience, pain tolerance would be increased.

I shall not discuss the psychophysics or physiology of pain but I will revert to some of the more mundane aspects of assessing pain for the purpose of evaluating the pain relieving attributes of drugs. At present we have no better measure of pain than the patients' reports of its presence and severity in their own words. If we will accept that there is some final common neural pathway for the subjective experience of pain, it is not unreasonable to assume that the effects of narcotics and other centrally acting analgesics can be validly assayed in this manner.

In a cancer hospital such as the one with which I am affiliated, finding patients with pain for which we can readily ascribe a cause is generally not too difficult. Those participating in our studies have been drawn from a fairly representative sample of our patient population with pain due either to their disease and its complications or to their treatment. Most in the latter category have been patients with self-limiting post-operative pain but in a significant number of cases there has been persistent pain after such procedures, among others, as chest all surgery and extensive radiation therapy to the brachial or lumbosacral plexus. Our research team nurse observers regularly examine the daily lists of patients scheduled for surgery and the medication records for patients receiving analgesics on all the adult floors of our hospital. Our data indicate that approximately 30 per cent of our patients, other than those with post-operative pain, receive analgesics for pain, and that about three out of four of these require narcotic type analgesics. Not all, of course, are suitable for our studies. The selection of patients for any study must be based on the objectives of the study and type of drugs or procedures which may be employed and, most importantly, on their appropriateness and safety in treating the patient-candidate, a determination which can be made by the research physicians only after examining the patient and/or the hospital chart.

### Nurse observers

Patients who are chosen and agree to participate in our studies are then seen at regular intervals by our nurse observers who record their observations on a daily pain chart (Fig. 2.1). The time at which the patient is seen and the site, quality and severity of pain are recorded at each interview (usually at hourly intervals) and entries are also made of unusual findings or events. When drugs are being evaluated, the nurse observer is supplied with sequentially number-coded test medications of uniform appearance and a non-study 'regular medication'. The latter is generally the known effective drug prescribed for the overnight and non-observation periods, and may be employed by the nurse should the patient require any analgesic in addition to the test medication during the observation period. Although the nurse observers

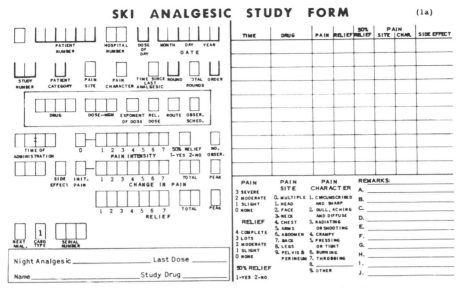

Fig. 2.1 Daily analgesic study form for recording fluctuations in pain and analgesic response to study medications and for ready conversion of data to punch cards for computer analysis.

are members of the analgesic studies research team and are not burdened with other duties of regular staff nurses, they are nonetheless fully qualified registered nurses and are expected to blend into the hospital medical care delivery system. Thus, the nurse observers have responsibilities to the regular staff nurses and physicians for detecting and reporting changes in the patient's status which may require attention whether or not they are in any conceivable way related to our studies. While they have been trained to avoid leading questions in their interviews and observations relating to our study objectives, our research nurses are alerted by the research team physician to potential or impending complications in the patient's medical condition and there have, in fact, been several instances in which our analgesic research nurses have been instrumental in the initiation of prompt medical attention when delays might have been disastrous. In keeping with this role, we have attempted to conduct our studies in a manner which is helpful rather than obtrusive to the regular staff and seems least out of the ordinary for the patient. It is in this kind of a setting that the patients' reports of pain are expected to be most meaningful for our investigations.

## Trial design

The majority of our studies and virtually all of our analgesic drug evaluations are conducted 'double-blind', employing some form of crossover design, appropriate standards and controls and randomisation of treatments,which are administered 'on demand' rather than by the clock (Wallenstein & Houde, 1975). An example of the type of data obtainable under these conditions is shown in Figure 2.2,the results of one of our earliest analgesic studies (Houde, Wallenstein & Rogers, 1960). In that particular study all the patients had chronic pain due to their disease, the majority from bone metastases. The measures of pain relief consisted of changes in

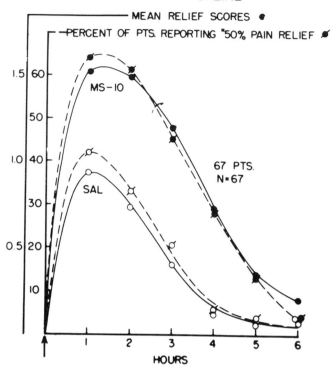

Fig. 2.2 Time-effect curves for morphine sulphate 10mg intramuscularly (dots) and sterile saline intramuscularly (circles) in terms of both the mean pain relief scores (solid lines) and the percentage of patients reporting at least 50 per cent relief of pain (broken lines) at each hour after medication. Each point represents the responses of the same 67 patients. (With permission of C.V. Mosby & Co, St. Louis).

pain intensity at each hourly postmedication observation period from the premedication value, utilising a four point categorical scale of from 'none' to 'severe' pain, and the number or percentage of patients who judged their pains 'at least half relieved' at each post-medication interview. Only a minority of patients actually obtained complete pain relief from either of the test medications, which were a 10 mg intramuscular dose of morphine and a sterile saline placebo. Not only was there a substantial placebo response but the time-effect curve mimicked that of morphine, although at a lower effect level, and the relative values of morphine and placebo were virtually the same by the two measures of pain relief — both based on intensity but expressed in quantitative terms in one case and in quantal terms in the other.


## Placebo response

Our subsequent experiences and those of other investigators have, of course, clearly documented that placebo responses are regularly encountered in circumstances under which the patient asks for medication that he has been led to expect will relieve his symptoms, as is the case generally when pain medication is requested. However, contrary to some statements in the medical literature, placebo response levels can vary appreciably from one population of patients to another and, in fact, from time to time in the same patients. It is therefore advisable when evaluating the effects and form of treatment on pain to include in the experimental design of each study some internal control or measure of the discriminatory ability of the method under those study conditions.

The variability among patients in analgesic scores after injections of morphine and a saline placebo is illustrated in Figure 2.3., a scatter diagram in which each of the 67 dots represents the six-hour total scores of a patient to each test medication. The

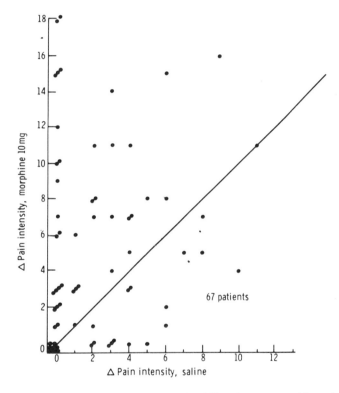

Fig. 2.3 Scatter diagram of the responses of each of 67 patients to morphine sulphate 10mg and sterile saline injection intramuscularly.

diagonal represents the line of no discrimination. The differences among patients in these terms are highly significant, which has been the case in virtually every analgesic study we have conducted over the course of the past 25 years. It is also worthy of note that while a sizeable proportion of patients reported some relief from placebo and a proportion of them even more relief from the saline injection than from morphine, we found it virtually impossible to screen out placebo reactors. The reason for this is that almost 90 per cent of our patients with unquestionable reasons for pain responded in some degree to placebo, if not at the original challenge, then when subsequently included in studies which included placebo controls. Many years ago Lasagna and his associates, working in Dr Beecher's laboratory in Boston, conducted

10

a study of placebo reactors and non-reactors who were subjected to a battery of psychological tests (Lasagna, *et al,* 1954) and found that the placebo reactors were those whom they characterised as the more normal. Non-reactors as a group were patients with more rigid personalities who tended to be suspicious of those caring for them and to fail to respond to any medication they were given.

A variety of circumstantial factors can influence placebo response and, as illustrated by our study of metopon, an analogue of morphine, one of these factors can be the effectiveness of other medications or treatments given for the same purposes (Fig. 2.4). This study was conducted as a series of sequentially related, graded dose,

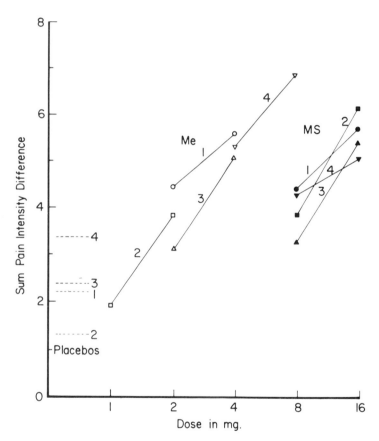

Fig. 2.4 Dose effect curves for intramuscular morphine (MS) and Metopon (Me). The changes in hourly pain intensity scores summed for 6 hours after medication (ordinate) are plotted against dose on a logarithmic scale (abscissa) for each of the four sequential experiments indicated by the numbers on the graph. Each study consists of an upper and lower dose of morphine (solid points) and of metopon (circles) connected by solid lines and a placebo plotted as a broken line.

double-blind experiments in several small groups of cancer patients with chronic pain, in which each patient received, in a randomised order, two doses of the standard drug, morphine, two doses of the test drug, metopon, and a sterile saline injection, all by intramuscular injection and on separate days. The results are plotted as drug-dose effect lines for each experiment (numbered successively), and the scores for the corresponding placebo as dashed horizontal lines. The doses of morphine, the standard drug, were kept the same but when the lower and less effective doses of metopon, the test drug, were given (series 2) the placebo scores were lower and *vice versa* (series 4). Graded doses of narcotic analgesics have been found quite consistently to produce graded analgesic responses in our study patient populations and, in general, this has also been true of my experience in titrating doses to each patient's needs in practice.

Analgesic drugs are, of course, not the only way, and sometimes they are not the appropriate way of treating pain — even that due to cancer. However, there is little question but that, in conjunction with the proper medical attention and evaluation which every patient in pain deserves to receive, they are by far the physician's most efficient means of contending with pain. Since, as I have mentioned above, graded doses of potent analgesics have given graded analgesic responses in patients with a large variety of painful states, the response to known doses of known analgesics may serve, in turn, as a means of assessing pain severity in clinical practice.

## Conclusion

Just over 15 years ago, I participated in a symposium in London (1961), sponsored by the Universities Federation for Animal Welfare, in which I spoke on the Assessment of Pain in Man, immediately after Drs H. Beecher and J.D. Hardy, who had somewhat divergent opinions on the subject. Taking advantage of my position in the order of speakers, I commented on their differences in terms of an allegorical reference to Alice in Wonderland which I had borrowed from an essay by Professor Durell (1956) on the Theory of Relativity and which I think is worthy of repetition. I likened the assessment of pain in man to a consideration of the geometry of Alice Through the Looking Glass (Lewis Carroll) for, I felt that, as onlookers, our Alice is revealed to us only through a looking-glass. Her size, indeed even her presence, are things that we can judge only by her reflected image, and though we do not know whether our looking glass is flat or curved, or even smooth or irregular, our problem is to determine whether, by experiment or artifice, we can hopefully define the real Alice's dimensions. My contentions were that although Beecher, the clinical pharmacologist, would have Alice stand up close to the looking-glass where her image would be readily discernible, and then have her drink of the Bottle which makes her smaller, Hardy, the physiologist, would have her stand so far back that her image would be too small to measure and then have her eat of the Cake which makes her larger. These two approaches to the problem were, in principle, quite similar — that of having Alice change her size so that the relative differences of her reflected proportions could be compared. I said then, that we may well never reach any agreement about Alice on an absolute scale, but we surely could on a relative scale, and I submitted that this was an equally valid way of characterising Alice. But alas, this may prove to be only of academic interest, for we now have Drs Kosterlitz, Hughes, Terenius, Goldstein, Pert, Snyder, Guillemin, Simon and a growing number of their colleagues who have discovered that, inherently, we all have morphine-like factors in our central nervous systems which seem to have something to do with pain. To assess pain perhaps all we will have to do is measure these factors.

## References

Bailey, C.A. & Davidson, P.O. (1976) The Language of Pain Intensity. *Pain,* 2, 319-324.
Beecher, H.K. (1959) *Measurements of Subjective Responses: Quantitative Effects of Drugs.* New York: Oxford University Press.
Durrell, C.V. (1956) The Theory of Relativity in *The World of Mathematics. Ed:* Newman, J.R. New York: Simon and Schuster. pp 1107-1114.
Houde, R.W., Wallenstein, S.L., & Rogers, A. (1960) Clinical Pharmacology of Analgesics: 1. A Method of Assaying Analgesic Effect. *Clinical Pharmacology and Therapeutics* 1, 163-174.
Houde, R.W., Wallenstein, S.L., & Beaver, W.T., (1966) Section vi, 1 Clinical Pharmacology International Executive of Pharmacologists and Therapeutists, London. Pergamon Press.
Keele, C.A. & Smith, R. (Eds) (1961) *Assessment of Pain in Man and Animals.* London and Edinburgh: Livingstone.
Lasagna, L., Mosteller, F., von Felsinger, J.M. & Beecher, H.K. (1954) A study of the Placebo Response. *American Journal of Medicine,* 16, 770-779.
Wallenstein, S.L. & Houde, R.W. (1975) Clinical Evaluation of Analgesic Effectiveness in: *Methods in Narcotic Research. Ed:* Ehrenpreis and Needle. New York: Marcel Dekker. pp 127-145.

# 3. The measurement of pain

M. ROSEN

Three aspects of pain measurement are considered; experimental or clinical studies of pain; a comparison of the accuracy of measurement; and comparision of doses of equal analgesic potency.

## Experimental or clinical measurement

1. In an experimental study, graduated stimuli can be applied double-blind and the response analysed by methods, such as signal detection analysis, which can examine the subject's willingness to report pain. Additional evidence about the sensitivity of the measurement can be obtained from the response to graduated doses of an analgesic drug,and a comparision between drugs can be arranged in crossover double-blind trials on volunteers. It is therefore possible to achieve a substantial degree of homogeneity in experimental design with trained volunteers and relatively reproducible results can be expected. The laboratory, however, does not truly mimic the clinical situation; the volunteer knows that the pain will be limited and so anxiety is decreased. Therefore it is essential to test analgesic drugs in the treatment of patients with real pain.
2. In clinical practice the pain stimulus is highly variable and may alter in character and degree unexpectedly. When comparing analgesic drugs, the treatment can be applied double-blind and patients can be adequately randomised,but it is only usually possible to arrange a crossover trial when studying chronic or terminal pain.

## Comparative accuracy of measurement

The patient's opinion of an analgesic is a synthesis of not only pain relief but also side effects, some desirable — euphoria or amnesia — others undesirable — nausea, dizziness, sedation or psychotomimetic effects. Under these difficult, and somewhat unreliable, circumstances it may seem reasonable to look for objective — if indirect — indications of pain, such as respiratory or hormonal changes produced by pain and which are assumed to be reversed by adequate pain relief. In any case, whether the measurement is subjective or objective, it is important to know the method's possible sensitivity and therefore power of discrimination (Table 3.1). Evidence is therefore required of the reproducibility of the measurement over the range under examination compared to the maximum discrimination (or change) that could occur with perfect pain relief and the degree of biological variation.

13

| Measurement of Pain | Reproducibility (95% Confidence Limits) | Discrimination | Notes: |
|---|---|---|---|
| **SUBJECTIVE** | | | |
| A. Grading:- | | | No. of grades limits sensitivity |
| None: Mild: Moderate: Severe | Narrow (probably) | 4 points | |
| B. Analogue Scale:- | | | |
| Visual Scale | 2% [1] | Infinite points | 1. Revill, et al (1976) |
| **OBJECTIVE (indirect)** | | | 1. Adams, et al (1967) |
| A. Ventilatory Measures:- | | | |
| (1) Arterial oxygen tension | 2% [1] | 24% [2] (5) | 2. % mean maximum change (sem) Spence and Smith (1975) |
| (2) Functional residual capacity | 8 – 16% [1] | 25% [2] (3) | 1. Cotes,(1975) |
| (3) Vital Capacity | | 70% [2] (8) | 2. % mean maximum change (sem) Spence and Smith, (1975) |
| B. Hormonal:- | | | 1. Huskisson, (1974) |
| Nor – adrenaline | 3% [1] | 30% [1,2] (40) | 2. % mean maximum change (sem) |

Table 3.1: A comparison between methods of measuring pain

### Subjective method

*Descriptive scale* Commonly the patient is asked to place pain into one or more grades such as 'none, mild, moderate or severe'. Alternatively, after treatment, pain-relief scales can be used as, 'no improvement, slight improvement, great improvement or pain-free'. If there are few grades — for instance, 'pain or no pain' — then it is likely that reporting of pain will be consistent, and it is reasonable to presume that reproducibility (95 per cent confidence limits) will be good. However, the maximum degree of discrimination cannot be more than the number of grades and the method can only have limited sensitivity.

*Visual analogue scale* Using unsegmented scales 10-20 centimetres in length, patients and subjects (18-35 years old) were asked to make a mark one-fifth along a line on ten consecutive occasions (Revill *et al,* 1976). The 95 per cent confidence limits were plus or minus 2 per cent of the full scale. Similarly, on a scale marked 'no pain' to 'as much as you can imagine' subjects were asked to mark the memory of a pain distant in time (toothache or dysmenorrhoea), and without warning to repeat the estimate 5 minutes and 24 hours after. The degree of accuracy was preserved; and also after pethidine 150 mg, which was somewhat surprising in a test which required visual and motor control. It would be advisable to repeat these checks before relying on the reproducibility of this method of reporting pain in other age groups and with other drugs.

Some analogue scales are segmented, which, by reducing the patient's choice, has a similar effect to a limited number of grades. Only a plain line can offer an infinite number of points with an unlimited choice of grade. It is impossible to know how many degrees of pain any particular patient can feel, although Hardy *et al.* (1952) considered that 21 grades of pain could be defined. The problem is somewhat academic since an unsegmented visual analogue will allow each subject to choose the maximum number of points that can personally be discriminated. Huskisson (1974) reported that the patients,when presented with both a linear analogue and a graded scale, tended to cluster their choice around the grades,and only 27 per cent used the whole extent of the analogue scale. However, it is not clear whether the scales were presented simultaneously or sequentially; if the former, the graded scale might have influenced patient's choice of analogue score.

The sensitivity (ratio of per cent maximum change in the measurement of confidence limits) of a subjective measurement can only be tested indirectly. For instance, the hourly mean analogue score has been recorded during labour up to full dilatation. Figure 3.1 indicates the response before delivery. There was a

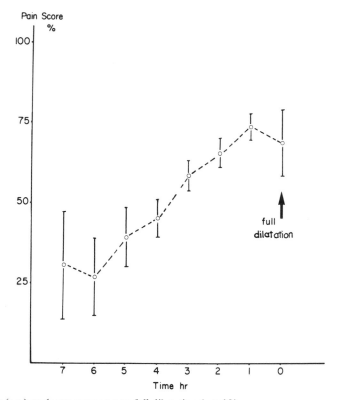

Fig. 3.1 Mean (s.e.) analogue scores up to full dilatation (n = 10)

change over a period of seven hours from a mean score of 25 per cent to 75 per cent of the maximum, and the score increases in an expected pattern closely paralleling cervical dilatation. This method seems to be reasonably sensitive at least for the measurement of severe pain.

### Objective methods
An objective measure can be used if there is a relationship between the measure and the relief of pain. Unfortunately there is a tendency to under-estimate limitations in reproducibility and discrimination of these measures.

*Respiratory measurements* Major changes in respiratory function occur after upper abdominal or thoracic operations and can be improved by adequate relief of pain. Nevertheless even perfect pain relief does not restore pre-operative respiratory function,so that the maximum effect of pain relief is limited.

Arterial oxygen tension can be measured within 5 per cent (95 per cent confidence limits) in most laboratories and even within 2 per cent (Adams, Morgan-Hughes, and Sykes, 1967). The mean fall in arterial oxygen tension after upper abdominal surgery from pre-operative values is about 25 per cent (Muneyuki *et al.*, 1968; Spence and Smith, 1971; Spence and Logan, 1975).

In laboratories which maintain high standards, most ventilatory tests have coefficients or variation in the range of 4-8 per cent (Cotes, 1975). In measures of functional residual capacity, or vital capacity, 95 per cent confidence limits within 16 per cent might be expected. After upper abdominal operations the mean change in FRC is about 25 per cent (Spence and Logan, 1975) so that this cannot be a very sensitive measure. Changes in vital capacity are larger and therefore should offer a more discriminating measure.

*Hormonal measurements* Excretion of catecholamines in urine has been measured in patients with rheumatoid arthritis treated with simple analgesics such as paracetamol or dextropropoxyphene. The 95 per cent confidence limits of the measurement of noradrenaline (at the concentrations found) were 15 per cent and the mean change in adrenaline secretion was about 40 per cent — so that this is a measure of limited sensitivity.

*Comparisons at equal potency*
It is important, although always difficult, to ensure that each drug is being tested at a dose capable of producing equal analgesia. The value of each drug can then be determined by comparing the incidence of desirable and undesirable side-effects. This problem causes great confusion in drug trials but can be avoided if the patient is allowed to determine the need and timing of each intravenous increment according to the pain felt, using an automatic patient-operated apparatus (Forrest, W.H. Jr., Smethurst, P.W. and Kienitz 1970; Evans *et al.*, 1976). In this way, when the patient is satisfied, demand is reduced by regulating the timing of the dose of analgesic, and the patient can obtain optimum pain relief (Fig. 3.2).

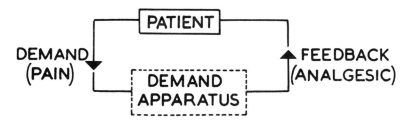

Fig. 3.2 Closed loop effect of pain relief on patient demand for analgesic

Furthermore, the patient's judgement is a balance of analgesia and side-effects, so that the practical value of each drug is being determined.

The Cardiff apparatus (Fig. 3.3) has a patient-operated push-button which

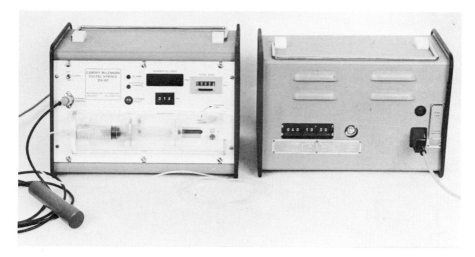

Fig. 3.3 Cardiff patient-operated demand apparatus

starts a syringe pump administering a fixed increment of drug to the patient
(McCarthy *et al.*, 1976. Evans *et al.*, 1976). An interval time-controller allows the
minimum period between increments to be set between 1 to 99 minutes. In obstetric
and post-operative trials this interval has been set at 10 minutes, which has proved
sufficient to enable both the increment to be administered slowly (3-4 mins) and
the patient to determine the effect. The syringe pump delivers a fixed volume but
an incremental dose (in micrograms) can be dialled directly with a thumb-switch
when a dilution factor is set. A display continuously indicates the residual amount
of the increment as it is being administered. Simultaneously, a separate counter
displays the accumulated total of drug administered. On the back of the machine,
behind a panel which can be locked, are controls to set the dilution factor, the
interval between increments, and the speed of injection.

In obstetric practice there were no significant differences between the means of
the total doses demanded when increments of pethidine varied between 0.125 mg/kg,
0.25 mg/kg, and 0.375 mg/kg. There is, therefore, evidence of feedback so that the
total dose demanded is related by the patient to increment size. This means that
the size of the increment need not be chosen precisely so long as it is not so small
that the patient can never be satisfied or so large as to cause undesirable side effects.
The system can easily be used in a double-blind trial. In practice, the apparatus can
be used under nursing supervision since the settings of the apparatus and the total
dose in the syringe are prescribed by the clinician in the same way as an intramuscular
injection.

In a pilot study (Sechzer, 1971) (under medical supervision) of pain relief after
upper abdominal surgery, 3 patients used the apparatus with pethidine and 5 with
buprenorphine. Figure 3.4 illustrates the pattern of demand of a patient who received
intravenous pethidine over 18 hours. In the immediate post-operative period the
mean dose demanded rose to nearly 2.7 mg/kg per hour, falling exponentially to
about 0.55 mg/kg/hour by the end of the period. The mean dose of pethidine
(46.4 mg) demanded per hour would compare reasonably with a duration of action

18

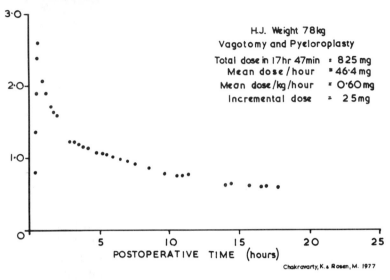

**PATIENT ACTIVATED ANALGESIC APPARATUS**

**PETHIDINE I.V.**

MEAN DOSE DURING
POSTOPERATIVE PERIOD (mg/kg/hr)

H.J. Weight 78kg
Vagotomy and Pyeloroplasty

Total dose in 17hr 47min = 825 mg
Mean dose/hour = 46·4 mg
Mean dose/kg/hour = 0·60 mg
Incremental dose = 2·5 mg

POSTOPERATIVE TIME (hours)

Chakravarty, K. & Rosen, M. 1977

Fig. 3.4 Use of Cardiff patient-activated apparatus with pethidine in a post-operative patient

of pethidine 100 mg intramuscularly of between 2 and 4 hours. It is unlikely however that the patient would have received the total dose administered (825 mg of pethidine) by any other method, although neither excessive sedation nor respiratory depression occurred.

Figure 3.5 shows a patient after a similar upper abdominal operation who demanded 0.65 μg/kg/hr buprenorphine in the immediate post-operative period, which rate fell to 0.3 μg/kg/hr towards the end of the 25 hour period. There was an increase in the demand rate between 5 and 12 hours and a long period of 13 hours when the patient made no demand. This pattern is unlike that with pethidine and may indicate that there were less unpleasant side effects.

Table 3.2 shows that the mean dose demanded of pethidine was 0.43 mg/kg/hr and of buprenorphine was 0.21 μg/kg/hr. The potency of buprenorphine compared to pethidine was therefore approximately 2000 to 1, which is a higher ratio than previously reported.

The measurement of pain remains difficult, but improvements in the sensitivity and discrimination of pain measurements could ensure satisfactory comparisions of treatment with smaller numbers of patients than previously possible.

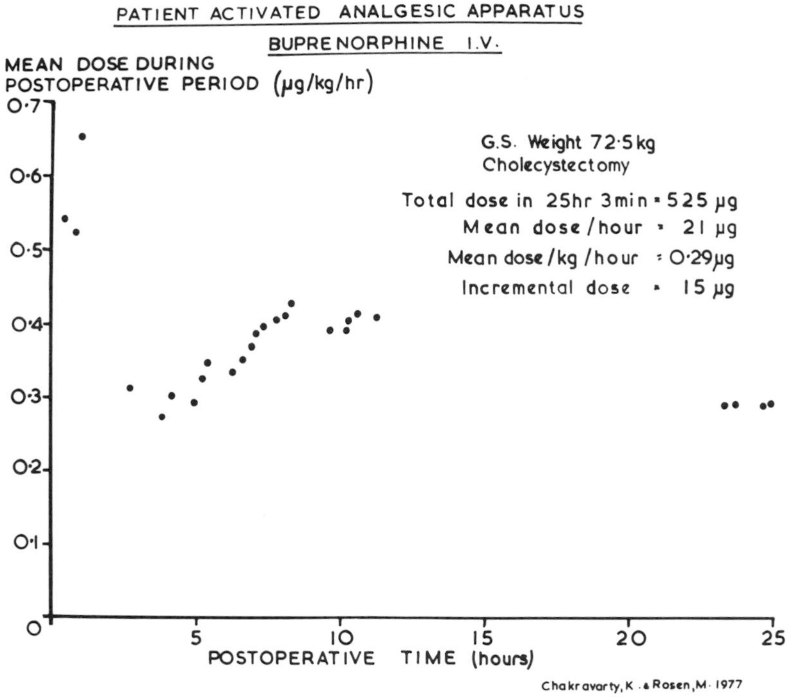
PATIENT ACTIVATED ANALGESIC APPARATUS
BUPRENORPHINE I.V.
MEAN DOSE DURING POSTOPERATIVE PERIOD (µg/kg/hr)
0·7
0·6
0·5
0·4
0·3
0·2
0·1
0
5
10
15
20
25
POSTOPERATIVE TIME (hours)
G.S. Weight 72·5 kg
Cholecystectomy
Total dose in 25hr 3min = 525 µg
Mean dose/hour = 21 µg
Mean dose/kg/hour = 0·29µg
Incremental dose = 15 µg
Chakravarty, K. & Rosen, M. 1977

Fig. 3.5 Use of Cardiff patient-activated apparatus with buprenorphine in a post-operative patient

| Patient | Sex | Weight (kg) | Duration of Analgesia (hours) | Total dose mg | mg/hr | mg/kg/hr |
|---|---|---|---|---|---|---|
| | | | PETHIDINE | | | |
| H. J. | M | 78 | 18 | 825 | 46.4 | 0.6 |
| M. S. | M | 66 | 13 | 435 | 33.04 | 0.5 |
| B. B. | F | 53 | 24 | 225 | 9.5 | 0.18 |
| | | | Mean | 495 | 29.6 | 0.43 |
| | | | BUPRENORPHINE | (ug) | ug/hr | ug/kg/hr |
| G. S. | F | 72.5 | 25 | 555 | 22.5 | 0.3 |
| C.B. | F | 67 | 20 | 315 | 15.3 | 0.2 |
| B. R. | F | 55.2 | 25 | 165 | 6.5 | 0.1 |
| L. R. | F | 71.75 | 22 | 525 | 23.6 | 0.3 |
| B. C. | F | 56.5 | 21 | 180 | 8.4 | 0.15 |
| | | | Mean | 348 | 15.26 | 0.21 |

Buprenorphine : Pethidine 1 : 2,000 (approx)

Table 3.2 Use of pethidine and buprenorphine in a pilot study of post-operative patients

20

**References**

Adams, A.P., Morgan-Hughes, J.O., and Sykes, M.K. (1967) pH and blood gas analysis. Methods of measurement and sources of error using electrode systems. *Anaesthesia, 22,* 575.

Cotes, J.E. (1975) *Lung Function: Assessment and Application in Medicine* 3rd Ed., Oxford: Blackwell.

Evans, J.M., McCarthy, J.P., Rosen, M. and Hogg, M.I.J. (1976) Apparatus for patient-controlled administration of intravenous narcotics during labour. *Lancet,* 1, 17.

Forrest, W.H.Jr., Smethurst, P.W.R., Kienitz, M.E., (1970) Self-administration of intravenous analgesics. *Anesthesiology,* 33, 363.

Hardy, J.D., Wolff, H.G. and Goodell, H. (1952) *Pain Sensations and Reactions,* Baltimore, Williams & Wilkins.

Huskisson, E.K. (1974) Catecholamine excretion and pain. *British Journal of Clinical Pharmacology,* 1, 80.

Huskisson, F.C. (1974) Measurement of pain. *Lancet,* 2, 1127.

McCarthy, J.P., Evans, J.M., Hogg, M.I.J., amd Rosen, M. (1976) Patient-controlled administration of intravenous analgesics. *Applications of Electronics in Medicine,* I.E.R.E. Conference Proceedings, Southampton.

Muneyuki, M., Ueda, Y., Urabe, N., Takeshita, H., and Inamoto, A. (1968) Postoperative pain relief and respiratory function in man. Comparison between intermittent intravenous injections of meperidine and continuous lumbar epidural analgesia. *Anesthesiology,* 29, 304.

Revill, S.I., Robinson, J.O., Rosen, M. and Hogg, M.I. (1976) The reliability of a linear analogue for evaluating pain. *Anaesthesia,* 31, 191.

Sechzer, P.H. (1971) Studies in pain with the analgesia-demand system. *Anesthesia and Analgesia* **50**: 1.

Spence, A.A. and Logan, D.A. (1975) Respiratory effects of extradural nerve block in the postoperative period. *British Journal of Anaesthesia,* 47, (Suppl.) 281.

Spence, A.A., and Smith, G. (1971) Postoperative analgesia and lung function: a comparison of morphine with extradural block. *British Journal of Anaesthesia,* 43, 144.

# 4. The interpretation of pain measurements

K. D. MACRAE

## Introduction

The need for pain measurement was clearly stated by Huskisson (1974).

> 'In clinical trials of drugs given for painful conditions, pain cannot be said to have been relieved unless it has been measured.'

However, whereas physical measurement, of length or weight for example, is intended and expected to give the same answer under varying background conditions, the measurement of a psychological experience such as pain presents a quite different set of problems. Consider, for example, the two lines AB and CD below. Although AB *appears* to be longer, CD is in fact *physically* longer. An observer who reports the

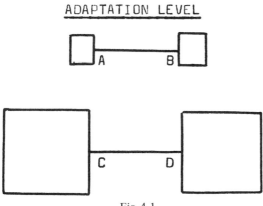

Fig. 4.1

*experience* that AB is longer is correctly reporting what he sees, even though this is at variance with the physical facts. Helson (1964), propounding his theory of perceptual relativity, states that the perception of any stimulus depends on the overall flux of energy received by the observer — perception is intrinsically relative.

A whole branch of psychology, known as psychophysics, is concerned with the relationship between physical quantities, such as size, brightness, or loudness, and their perception. In the measurement of pain, however, there is no suitable physical stimulus to measure, except in the case of experimentally induced pain, and there remains the problem of measuring a private perception. Again, it is appropriate to quote Huskisson (1974).

'Pain is a personal psychological experience, and an observer can play no legitimate part in its direct measurement.'

### The measurement of pain

How, then, has the problem of the measurement of pain been approached? The most obvious, and most used, method is to ask for the directly reported experience of the observer, who describes the amount of pain he feels on some scale. It is on this approach that the present discussion will largely concentrate. However, other methods have been used, including such indirect methods as measuring vital capacity or demands for analgesia. Observers have attempted to assess the degree of pain felt by others, and the matching of pathological pain with experimentally induced pain has also been studied.

Returning to measurement of pain by directly reported experience, the simplest form of measurement is a *qualitative scale,* where the observer simply reports whether the pain is absent or present. A potentially more sensitive assessment can be attempted by asking the observer to grade his pain into *ordered categories,* such as mild, moderate and severe. If, as Huskisson (1974) suggests, pain relief is also measured, the ordered categories could be none, slight, moderate and complete. Increased sensitivity comes up against the limits of the English language, and this is overcome by the use of multi-point numerical scales, such as can be obtained from visual *analogue scales.*

Although these scales are in ascending order of sensitivity, their usefulness depends on two other properties, namely reliability and validity.

### *Reliability*

Reliability results from the absence of random or systematic error. It is obviously impossible to achieve the complete absence of error in any measurement process, physical or psychological, but the important requirement is that the error be small in relation to the use made of the measurements.

A simple check on reliability can be provided by an immediate re-test to check how consistently the observer reports his pain perception. Longer-term reliability is much more difficult to assess, as this requires the assumption that the level of pain experience was constant over the time interval involved.

Reliability and sensitivity are to some extent in conflict, as the more sensitive the scale the more noticeable will small degrees of unreliability be. The primary requirement is as stated above, that the error be small in relation to the changes being measured — e.g. as a result of treatment.

### *Validity*

Validity is a much more difficult property to establish, as the very nature and meaning of the measurement is in question. With a simple physical measurement validity may not be a problem, as there can be little doubt about what is being measured. However, with a private experience such as pain there is an immediate and important question about whether we are measuring what we wish to measure.

The validity of a measurement process can be considered in at least four ways. First, the *face validity* of the measurement can be assessed, by finding if the measuring instrument appears to a naive observer, such as a patient, to be a sensible way of measuring the quantity in question. This is, of course, neither a necessary nor a sufficient form of validity, in that a good measurement may not be an obvious one, nor an obvious one a good one. Secondly, the measuring instrument can be assessed by a number of 'expert' judges in order to ascertain whether it has *content validity*. That the measuring instrument was designed by such an 'expert' in the first place is of course relevant in this respect, but it is best to have the content validity judged by a number of experts independently of each other. Thirdly, if it is possible to correlate the measurement of pain with one or more external criteria an assessment of the *concurrent validity* of the scale can be made. With experimentally induced pain it would be expected that as the intensity of the pain-provoking stimulus increased the reported perception of pain would also show an increase. The difficulty with concurrent validity is in finding a criterion against which to assess the measurement in question, as it is all too possible that apparent validity is based on a totally circular argument. Fourthly and finally, there is *construct validity*, which is described in detail by Cronbach (1960). Construct validity is concerned with how our theoretical understanding of the construct being measured (here it is pain) relates to experimental findings. Thus, for example, it might be expected that as the wound resulting from a surgical operation heals, the level of pain experienced will decrease, or that, as pain in an arthritic joint is relieved, there will be a lessening of functional impairment. As Kerlinger (1964) points out, whenever an hypothesis is tested or relationships are empirically examined, construct validity is involved. Construct validity therefore includes aspects of face, content and concurrent validity.

### Interpretation of the measurements

Finally, there is the problem of the meaning of the numbers resulting from pain measurement. With a simple qualitative scale, in which we can denote pain absent by 0 and pain present by 1, an absolute threshold for pain perception is being assessed. The observer simply requires the capacity to distinguish between the presence and absence of pain; but even if complete reliability were to be (falsely) assumed, the sensitivity of this measurement is inadequate for most purposes.

When the observer is asked to grade his pain into ordered categories, none as 0, mild as 1, moderate as 2 and severe as 3 for instance, there is now a requirement for the ability to discriminate between three degrees of actual pain in addition to determining the presence or absence of it. The sensitivity of this scale is somewhat limited, and the question also arises about the equality of the intervals in the scale. Is the change from 1 to 2 of equal magnitude to the change from 2 to 3?

An increase in sensitivity has, as we have seen, been sought through the use of the visual analogue scale, in which a 100 mm line is commonly used. The perception of pain can be expressed as a distance from 0 in 1 mm steps, or some coarser grouping maybe used — 20 intervals of 5 mm, for example. The increase in sensitivity may well have been bought at the expense of some apparent unreliability — whether the

24

reliability is acceptable requires investigation. Aitken (1969) has suggested that analogue scales are subjected to the arcsine transformation in order to reduce any skewness and produce an 'improvement towards normality'. Such a transformation has implications for the meaning of a change of a given amount, say 10 mm, between two judgments of pain intensity. Is a change from 0 to 10 mm equal in magnitude to a change from 40 to 50 mm? The effect of the arcsine transformation $(X = \arcsin\sqrt{X})$ on a uniform distribution is shown below.

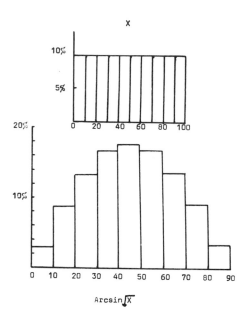

Fig. 4.2 The effect of the arcsine transformation on a uniform distribution.

It is clear that the effect of the transformation is to stretch the ends of the scale in comparison with the middle. To further illustrate this point, the distance 0 to 10 mm transforms to a change of 18.4, the distance 10 to 20 mm transforms to 8.2, and the distance 40 to 50 mm to 5.8. Thus, the arcsine transformation makes changes in reported pain on the raw scale greater at the extremes of the scale than in the middle. Although this does produce an 'improvement towards normality', the question still remains whether this is a more realistic scaling of the pain than the original scale.

References

Aitken, R.C.B. (1969) Measurement of feelings using visual analogue scales. *Proceedings of the Royal Society of Medicine*, **62**, 989-993.
Cronbach, L. (1960) *Essentials of Psychological Testing*, 2nd Ed. New York: Harper and Row.
Helson, H. (1964) *Adaptation-level Theory*. New York: Harper and Row.
Huskisson, E.C. (1974) Measurement of pain. *Lancet*, **2** 1127-1131.
Kerlinger, F.N. (1964) *Foundations of Behavioural Reasearch*. New York: Holt, Rinehart and Winston.

## Discussion

*Session 1*
*Mr Rosenfeldt.* Is median sternotomy a painful incision if reconstituted correctly?
*Prof. Donald.* I can compare both median sternotomy and lateral thoracotomy incisions and certainly the mid-sternal split was the more painful.
*Dr Clarke.* Does the pain last long into the post-operative period?
*Prof. Donald.* In my case pain lasted for about 10 days.
*Dr Clarke.* How does a thoracic incision compare with that of laparotomy?
*Prof. Donald.* I found thoracotomy much more painful than laparotomy.
*Prof. Hobbs.* What was the effect of analgesic drugs on severe pain, Professor Donald, and what do you consider was of most help in controlling your pain?
*Prof. Donald.* The value of analgesics was unquestionably great, although appreciation of their value was lessened by the amnesia which they induced. I believe that psychological attitudes are of tremendous importance and careful psychological preparation before submission to any painful procedure allows more ready acceptance of what is going on and any treatment that is prescribed. It helps, of course, to know that the condition is curable.

*Dr Houde.* My experience with patients in chronic pain is different from that with severe acute pain. Careful preparation is just as important, but the patient must be able to function under the influence of medication.
*Dr Raftery.* Does Dr Houde think that factors such as social integration, interest in outside events, appetite and mobility should be used in the measurement of clinical response to the treatment of chronic pain?
*Dr Houde.* They are important factors in the management of patients but in experimental measurement we exclude these variables by studies designed to use each patient as his or her own control.
*Dr Rosen.* I endorse the comments about the importance of psychological attitudes. If, in practice, analgesics are not given promptly or in adequate amounts during the post-operative period, the patient's fear is enhanced, rendering any pain therapy less effective. This stems from the fear held by many physicians that dependence may be induced.
*Dr Masson.* I think we underestimate the safety of morphine and would suggest that even in widespread clinical use, dangerous overdosage is rare.
*Dr Alexander.* In a study of two groups of patients we found that the majority of patients in the group given 10 mg morphine/70 kg on demand (mean no. of injections 2.6/24 hours) had persistent or recurrent pain, whereas only one patient had persistent pain in the group given morphine 10 mg/70 kg every four hours.

Carbon dioxide tension was higher in the latter group but the rises remained within the physiological range in both groups, demonstrating that with adequate analgesia, ventilation is not necessarily depressed. This was further demonstrated by the small difference in arterial $PO_2$ levels between the groups with a marked difference in pain relief.
*Dr Raftery.* Is 10 mg morphine sufficient to act as a standard reference dose of analgesic?

*Dr Houde.* Fundamentally, the dose must be adequate to meet the situation and we use doses of morphine between 8 mg and 16 mg. It is important however, that sustained analgesia from repeated dose regimens should not encourage the medical care delivery team to become complacent.

*Dr Alexander.* This is much less of a problem with analgesics than with regional techniques such as epidural block. New symptoms which may be missed with epidural block will probably not be masked by analgesic agents.

*Dr Scoular.* Severe pain is interpreted by each patient in a different way. How does this affect the use of analogue scales?

*Dr Alexander.* The minimal requirement of drug assessment must be that the measurement is not influenced by the measuring technique and that the random error is not an appreciable part of the final dimension.

A further problem is that we are using different points for comparison. As an example, following pre-tibial compression the greater the pressure the greater the pain (experimental pain). Using the hot lamp technique, as the lamp approaches the skin, the pain increases and then rises exponentially. However, with low back pain, for example, marked degrees can be tolerated and then suddenly the pain becomes unbearable. If these pains are measured on a linear analogue scale how can we be certain that any real difference is being measured? Does an interval of 10 per cent on an analogue scale actually represent a difference of 10 per cent in pain intensity?

Using the unmarked standard pain chart of 0-100 per cent against time, one finds that pain varies widely in the same patient, with peaks of intensity which are not reflected by the mean.

In the pain of ischaemic heart disease, three types of pain namely constant soreness, left and right sided angina can be identified using this method, but would not be apparent on a single-reading linear analogue scale. I believe that a disability score of essential activities such as breathing, washing or shaving offers a more realistic approach to pain assessment than linear analogue scales or disability scores which depend on voluntary activities.

*Dr MacRae.* The influence of measuring techniques on the perception of pain will not affect the final outcome because if similar groups are compared the same bias will be applied to each.

*Dr Rosen.* This is the whole basis of properly prepared controlled clinical trials, which must always be undertaken to elicit the true identity of any new compound.

# Session 2  Chairman: R. W. Houde

# 5. Analgesics and ureteral function

G S WATSON AND P EDMOND

Renal colic, or more accurately, ureteral colic is due to an increase in the intraluminal pressure which results in the ureteric muscle being stretched and possibly becoming ischaemic. Pain from the ureter is referred to the eleventh and twelfth thoracic somatic segments and the first lumbar segment. The pain may be severe and is most commonly evoked by a calculus. In these patients, where a definite cause is shown, the localisation and type of pain may be monitored during the passage of the causative agent. The patient, however, may require analgesics to be given usually on an arbitrary basis, often in increasing doses without primary consideration of the effect of the analgesic agent on either the kidney, as evidenced by any drug causing a fall in blood pressure, thereby affecting glomerular filtration, or by any consideration of a direct effect on ureteral function itself. The primary stimulus to ureteral contraction is a change in volume of the fluid content and therefore the activity may be altered by increasing the content (Lapides 1948). Although pain may be referred via the somatic segments, denervation of the ureter does not impair function, nor reduce the ability of the ureter to respond to change in urine volume.

Ureteral function has been studied during the course of routine retrograde pyelography using an established clinical technique designed to ensure that the intact organ in the intact patient is studied (Ross and Edmond 1965).

In this technique, the ureteral catheter is linked to a pressure transducer and complexes are recorded on a multichannel recorder. These complexes are considered to be due to the pressure changes within the renal pelvis and ureter consequent to the muscular contraction of the wall. They also give a reproducible indication of ureteral function. The recordings presented have been made under general anaesthesia. Anaesthetic agents may affect renal function but Kiil (1957) and subsequently Ross *et al* (1972) observed that recordings under general anaesthetic did not differ from those on the unanaesthetised subject. Although an indwelling ureteral catheter must introduce an abnormal factor in the assessment of ureteral function, provided that the catheter is non-occlusive it has been shown not to affect peristalsis to any appreciable extent when compared with observations from cinefluography or external monitoring techniques. (Fig. 5.1).

It is important to know that the pressure changes are those occurring at the catheter tip. To define the site of the contraction, the methodology has been confirmed by obtaining a simultaneous recording of the local action potential (EMG), using a double platinum electrode and recording EMG and pressure simultaneously (Ross *et al,* 1972).

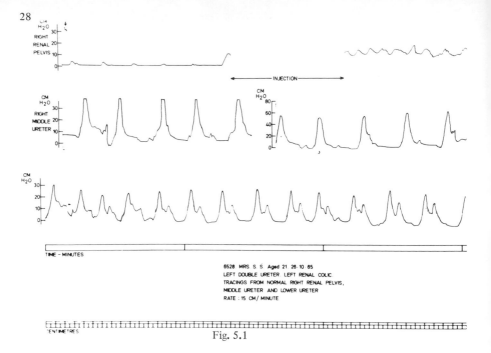

Fig. 5.1

Thus the technique offers a means of measuring the ureteral activity under physiological conditions (Figs. 5.2 and 5.3) and may be used to assess the speed and extent of activity of antispasmodic and analgesic drugs. Respiratory and vascular pulsation

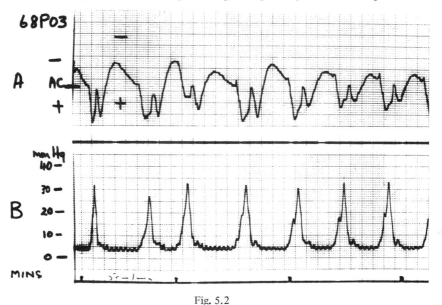

Fig. 5.2

may effect the ureteral recordings. The respiratory component may be eliminated by evoking a period of apnoea. This also indicates that the record obtained in the conscious patient is similar to that obtained from the anaesthetised subject.

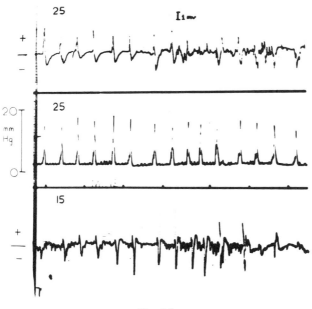

Fig. 5.3

The vascular components are small irregular waves seen only during the period of apnoea (Fig. 5.4). Before the effects of analgesics and antispasmodics are assessed a review of the normal observations will be made.

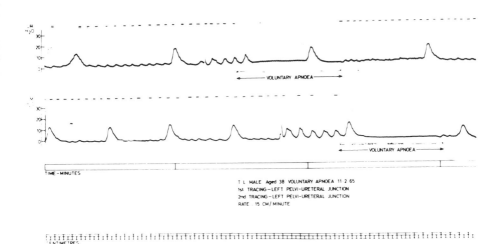

Fig. 5.4

## Rate of contraction

The ureteral contraction is regular and averages three per minute in the lower ureter. The rate is influenced by injection of fluid into the ureter — a technique to simulate increasing urinary flow.

## Rhythm

In the normal healthy ureter there is marked regularity of rhythm in the contraction waves, usually a single phase wave occurring at regular intervals. In the lower third of the ureter a diphasic form may be seen but, for each individual, this is often a constant feature (Fig. 5.5).

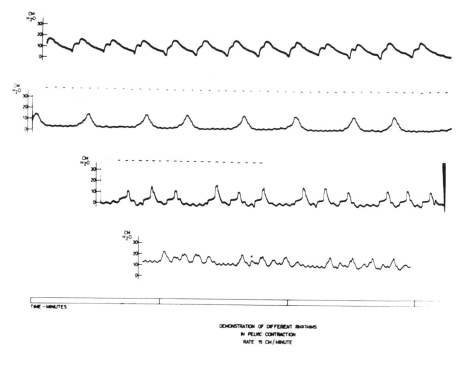

Fig. 5.5

## Amplitude

The ureteral contractions in the upper and middle third have an average height of 40 cm of water with a duration of seven seconds.

## Bilateral observations

Simultaneous recordings from both ureters demonstrate that the ureters do not contract synchronously. However, alteration in the rhythm extending to complete cessation of activity can ensue following the filling of the opposite renal pelvis.

The relationship of ureteral function to the autonomic nervous system is not fully understood. The ureteral nerves are arranged in superior, mid and inferior groups (Risholm, 1954). These nerves form a rich network of nerve fibres in the adventitia of the ureter. Electronmicroscopic studies of the ureter have shown numerous nerve bundles in the adventitious outer layer, either scattered randomly in this layer or partially interleaved with the most superficial muscle cells (Notley 1968, 1969, 1970).

These nerves are unmyelinated, but no true ganglion cells are identified. The conduction of action potential from cell to cell is considered to be due to the spread of action current around the intercellular space in overlapping muscle cells, no nerve plexus being involved. However, there is definite evidence that in man and in animal there is a degree of nervous control over peristalsis. The nervous system does integrate function of the left and right urinary tracts and may be responsible for reflex anuria seen occasionally (Ross *et al*, 1972).

With this base line information, we can now consider the action of drugs. It is well known that antispasmodic drugs are beneficial in the relief of ureteral colic, but evidence as to their action has been controversial (Kiil 1957, Hanley, 1953). However, in general the discrepancy in results has been due either to a failure to employ sufficiently sensitive apparatus, or to a failure to recognise the influence of circulatory changes on the urine production.

We have demonstrated that atropine, probanthine, hyoscine n-butyl bromide (Buscopan) and also the strong analgesics, morphine, omnopon and pethidine, all may have a depressant effect on ureteral peristalsis (Ross, Edmond and Griffiths, 1967). The effects are a slowing of the rate of contraction, producing irregularity of rhythm and reducing the amplitude of the contraction, while altering the form of the contraction waves (Figs. 5.6 and 5.7). There is a considerable patient variable as to the time response, which is not due to difference in dosage per body weight alone.

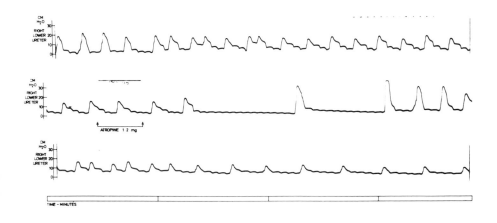

Fig. 5.6

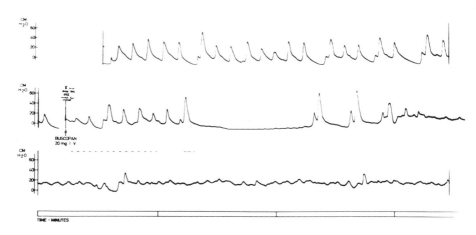

Fig. 5.7

The effects of antispasmodics are fairly brief and this should be considered in the clinical administration. Their action is due to a local effect not mediated purely by alteration in the circulatory activity. In the search for the perfect analgesic, a drug to relax the ureter between contractions must be considered, although it should be borne in mind that a dilated ureter provides an inefficient transport system for fluid or for a foreign body.

The criteria for the perfect analgesic in the relief of ureteral colic must therefore include the following:

Firstly, it should relieve pain rapidly. Secondly, it should continue, or even increase peristaltic activity to allow the calculus to pass down the ureter more rapidly, yet without causing any transient muscle ischaemia. However, these two factors may be mutually exclusive. The potent analgesics and those commonly administered anti-cholinergic drugs act by depressing ureteral peristalsis and therefore may actually delay any movement of the calculus. It has been shown that an increased fluid output is in itself a factor which may increase the peristaltic activity of the ureter, but to allow this, the third factor required is that the drug must have little effect on the circulation. Fourthly, it should not cause nausea or vomiting, which would decrease fluid intake, or increase fluid loss.

In summary, therefore, when assessing the efficiency of an analgesic to relieve pain of ureteral colic, due consideration should be given to the function of the ureters themselves. Should we maintain or increase peristalis, which may assist the passage of the calculus, at the risk of inducing muscle ischaemia, and possibly extravasation of urine? Or should we depress ureteral activity, allow the ureter to dilate and become an inefficient contractile organ, diminishing the chance of spontaneous movement of the offending calculus?

Ureteral colic is a common medical emergency demanding urgent treatment. The techniques for the direct measurement of the effects of available drugs, either analgesics, antispasmodics or even spasmodics, are now available and it is hoped that these studies will lead to a better understanding of the management of these patients.

## References

Hanley, H.G. (1953) *British Journal of Urology, 25*, 358.
Kiil, F. (1957) The function of the Ureter and Renal Pelvis. Philadelphia: W.B. Saunders Co.
Lapides, J. (1948) *Journal of Urology, 59*, 501.
Notley, R.G. (1968) Electron microscopy of the upper ureter and the pelvic – ureteric junction. *British Journal of Urology, 40*, 37-52.
Notley, R.G. (1969) The innervation of the upper ureter in man and in the rat: an ultrastructural study. *Journal of Anatomy, 105*, 393-402.
Notley, R.G. (1970) Calyceal obstruction due to parapelvic cyst. *British Journal of Urology, 42*, 439-445.
Risholm, L. (1954) *Acta Chirurgica Scandinavica, 107*, 599-600.
Ross, J.A,, Edmond, P. and Coull, J. (1965) The 'dynamic function' of the intact human renal pelvis and ureter. *British Journal of Surgery, 52*, 617-621.
Ross, J.A., Edmond, P. and Griffiths, J.M. (1967) The action of drugs on the intact human ureter. *British Journal of Urology, 39*, 26-30.
Ross, J.A., Edmond, P. and Kirkland, J.S. (1972) *Behaviour of the Human Ureter in Health and Disease.* Edinburgh and London: Churchill Livingstone.

# 6. Respiratory effects of strong analgesics

SHEILA JENNETT

The obvious questions which we want to ask about any strong analgesic drug are firstly, does it in fact cause respiratory depression; secondly, what is the magnitude and the time course of that depression in relation to the effectiveness of analgesia; and thirdly, if there is depression is it of any significance in the clinical situations in which the analgesic is going to be used. I shall be dealing mainly with the first two of these, not because they are the most important, but because they are widely studied and I have been involved in such studies myself.

If a drug decreases ventilation, it does not necessarily cause respiratory depression (Fig. 6.1). One has first to rule out the possibility of there being a relief of pain,

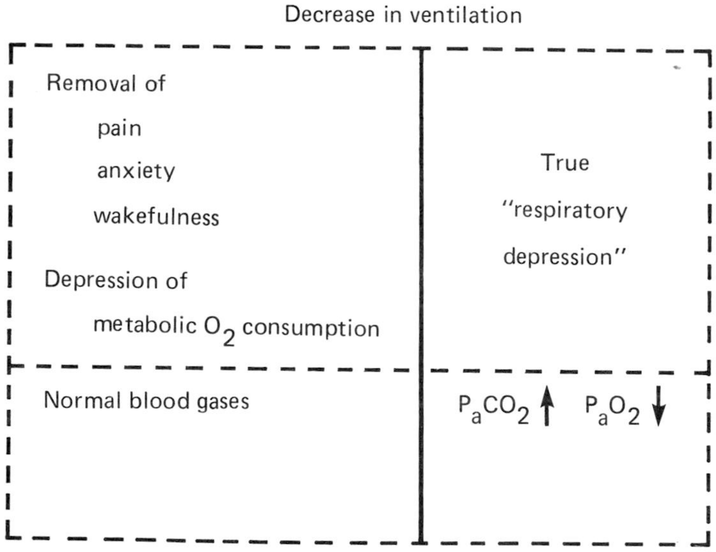

Decrease in ventilation

| Removal of | True |
| pain | "respiratory |
| anxiety | depression" |
| wakefulness | |
| Depression of | |
| metabolic $O_2$ consumption | |
| Normal blood gases | $P_aCO_2 \uparrow$   $P_aO_2 \downarrow$ |

Fig. 6.1

anxiety or wakefulness, any of which would be contributing to the respiratory drive. The second thing which is perhaps less often remembered is that the drug may be causing metabolic depression, reducing the requirement for ventilation, so that a decrease is appropriate; only if these are ruled out can we say that there is genuine respiratory depression.

The difference between these categories of decreased ventilation would be that in true respiratory depression there would be a tendency to hypercapnia and hypoxia and in the other conditions the blood gases would probably be normal. Drugs which are effective analgesics may have both these effects.

It has been shown that narcotic analgesics do decrease metabolic oxygen consumption as well as depressing the respiratory centres, and so the decrease in ventilation is the sum of these two effects. For example, in some studies of our own (Jennett, Barker & Forrest, 1968) comparing phenoperidine, pentazocine and morphine, there was a decrease in ventilation which was not so very different between these drugs. But there was a greater decrease with the phenoperidine initially which was disproportionately greater than the increase in $PCO_2$, because this drug decreased the metabolic oxygen requirement rather more than the others (compare a, b, c, Fig. 6.2).

It would appear from the literature that in general all analgesics which have been compared at approximately equi-analgesic doses show very similar respiratory depressant effects at around the usual effective dose. The respects in which the drugs *differ* are:-

1. In producing a peak effect at different times after administration
2. In the dose-response relationship.

One example of such differences is shown (Fig. 6.3). When we gave two consecutive relatively small doses of pethidine, there was a continually increasing depression. When we gave two relatively small consecutive doses of pentazocine there was not only a failure to produce further depression of ventilation, but it even increased a little. When we gave twice that dose all at once, both drugs caused a similar depression, but the recovery was quicker with pentazocine. So the points to be taken from this comparison are that the pethidine showed a relatively proportional dose-response, in that the double dose caused a double effect; the pentazocine did not show this, and also showed a more rapid recovery (Engineer and Jennett, 1972). The presence of a 'ceiling effect' has been shown for the narcotic antagonist group of analgesics; significant work on this has been done by Smith and his group in Philadelphia who have shown that there is a point at a dose equi-analgesic with about 0.4 mg/kg of morphine, at which pentazocine and related drugs will cease to cause further respiratory depression as the dose increases (Smith, 1971). Whether or not buprenorphine reaches such a ceiling I think still remains to be demonstrated (see Orwin, Orwin & Price, 1976); this clearly can be of significance; if the respiratory depression is significant at all, we want to know whether increasing dosage will increase the depression.

I have avoided the question of how we are defining the extent of a respiratory depression. The examples so far were in terms of air-breathing changes: rise in $PCO_2$ and decrease in ventilation. From time to time I have defended this relatively simple measurement as an estimate of respiratory depression, partly on account of the coefficients of variation for different estimations. I should like to think that variability between repeated measurements is not always related to the standard of the laboratory but also perhaps to some *real* variation in some of the factors which are measured. When we did a series of repeated measurements on normal subjects, we found that ventilation and $P_aCO_2$ varied relatively little compared to the parameters of the $CO_2$ response (Jennett, 1968). For this reason, we demonstrated a greater statistical significance in the changes after a drug in the $PCO_2$ and in the ventilation than we did

36

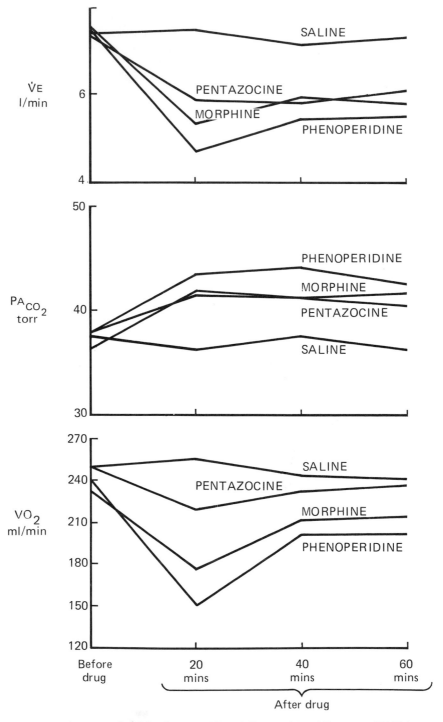

(pentazocine 20, phenoperidine 1.5, morphine 10 mg per 70 Kg)

Fig. 6.2 Changes in the extent and pattern of ventilation, $P_aCO_2$ and oxygen consumption in six subjects

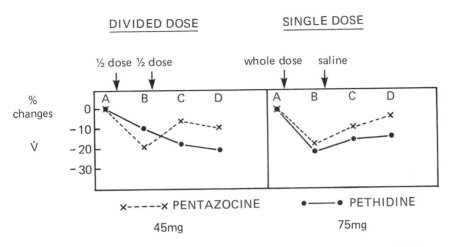

Fig. 6.3 The effect of single and repeated doses of pentazocine and pethidine on ventilation.

in the parameters of the $CO_2$ response (Jennett *et al.*, 1968). However, having said that, $CO_2$ responses are the tests which are most often and very widely done in order to estimate respiratory depressant effects, despite many published and unpublished reports of poor repeatability (see Jennett, 1976).

The type of test which is very commonly done now, because it is brief and therefore well-suited to consecutive measurements, is some form of re-breathing test. A small volume of gas is re-breathed, starting at 5-7 per cent $CO_2$, the $PCO_2$ rises linearly, the ventilation rises approximately linearly, and many points can be obtained from a 3-minute recording in order to plot a response line (Read, 1967).

When response lines are plotted, different treatments of data are applied in order to describe what has happened as a result of drug administration; and there are a great many different ways of describing the $CO_2$ responses, as well as a great many methods of carrying them out. Two types of change can occur (Fig. 6.4); a parallel shift

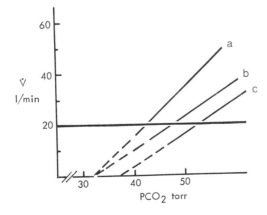

Fig. 6.4 $CO_2$ response lines showing parallel shift and change in slope.

or a change in slope. It has become the widely accepted practice in the literature of drug assessment to quote the displacement of the response curve at 20 litres per minute of ventilation. However, a similar 'displacement' value could mean that there is either a decrease in slope (A − B), or a shift to the right (B − C), or both. So this parameter on its own does not distinguish between the two sorts of change. Even if it does not, does it matter as long as it is a reproducible index of respiratory depression? I suggest that it *may* matter from the point of view of trying to define the site of action of these drugs, which could in turn have some eventual significance in relation to the clinical situations in which they are used.

In control system terms, the distinction is between altering the set point and altering the gain of the system. In physiological terms 'shift' and 'slope' changes could mean differences in the site or in the mechanism of action. It is generally assumed that respiratory depressant drugs act on the ponto-medullary centres. This is a reasonable assumption because they are known to act in other ways in the central nervous system. But the direct evidence that this is where they act on respiration is not very extensive. The fact that the respiratory pattern may be altered quite considerably, even when the response to rising $CO_2$ and the air-breathing $PCO_2$ are relatively unaffected, seems to be one of the best pieces of evidence that the computation of volume and frequency within the respiratory centres is one of the major things which are affected. But there are other possible sites of action (Fig. 6.5). If one is testing the response of the system to the challenge of high $CO_2$ in high oxygen then the response could be blunted either at the level of the medullary chemoreceptors or at the ponto-medullary centres themselves; hyperoxia excludes a peripheral chemoreflex effect. A difference in the site of action could matter in that, if the centres themselves were relatively undepressed, then they could be better stimulated by factors other than $CO_2$, such as agents which stimulate the arterial chemoreceptors.

It is also possible that the drug which depresses respiration might be affecting the arterial chemoreceptors (Fig. 6.5). As far as I am aware this remains relatively or

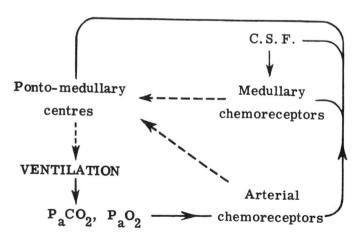

Chemical feedback via blood ( ⟶ )
and neural pathways ( --➤ )

Fig. 6.5.

completely unexplored. There have been studies on anaesthetic drugs in this context but not on analgesic drugs. Again, could this be important? It seems that it could, because there is not infrequently a hazard of hypoxia so that an inability to respond to hypoxia could be a serious disability in post-operative situations. If it is the centres themselves which are depressed, then, of course, there will be a depressed chemoreflex response to hypoxia as well as to $CO_2$.

It is perhaps not surprising that the response to hypoxia after analgesic drugs has been studied so very much less than the response to high $CO_2$. This stems from the assumption that it is the respiratory centres that are the depressed area, and it is also related to the relative difficulty of measuring the response to hypoxia. But there has been a recent report from Weil's group in Denver who have studied the ventilatory response to hypoxia very extensively in other situations. They control the $PCO_2$ at a steady level so that alterations in the $CO_2$- stimulus do not interfere with the situation, and steadily reduce the oxygen tension in the inspired air; the ventilation goes up eventually when oxygen tension gets to around 60 torr, and they can plot ventilation against $PO_2$. They have now studied this response after morphine, and they show that instead of the normal curve they get a very considerable depression (Weil *et al*, 1975). That might appear to suggest that there is an arterial chemoreceptor depression, but, in fact, in the same subjects they found also a diminished response to $CO_2$ in oxygen. Thus they were producing evidence that the depression is essentially in the medullary centres themselves.

The third question is whether any depression which does occur is going to be significant in the situations in which the drugs are used. Analgesic drugs have been shown to have a greater effect in reducing ventilation when the drug is given during an anaesthetic than when it is given to a normal conscious person (Table 6.1).

|  | Conscious subjects (Engineer and Jennett, 1972) | | Anaesthetized subjects (Davie, Scott and Stephen, 1970) | |
|---|---|---|---|---|
|  | Dose (mg) | Mean maximal reduction in $\dot{V}$ (%) | Dose (mg) | Mean maximal reduction in $\dot{V}$ (%) |
| Pentazocine | 22.5 | 19 | 30 | 67 |
|  | 45 | 18 |  |  |
| Pethidine | 37.5 | 9 | 30 | 41 |
|  | 75 | 21 |  |  |

Table 6.1 Effect of analgesics on ventilation in conscious and anaesthetised subjects.

Post-operatively this can be of significance. Otherwise we have already seen evidence that probably, in most clinical circumstances, the degree of depression is not important in relation to the effectiveness of analgesia.

I have been as impressed as anyone with the fact that narcotic analgesics can *improve*

40

ventilation and even improve the arterial oxygen tension when breathing is made easier by relieving pain.

## References

Davie, I.T., Scott, D.B. and Stephen, G.W. (1970) Respiratory effects of pentazocine and pethidine in patients anaesthetised with halothane and oxygen. *British Journal of Anaesthesia* **42**: 113-118.

Engineer, S. and Jennett, S. (1972) Respiratory depression following single and repeated doses of pentazocine and pethidine. *British Journal of Anaesthesia* **44**: 795-802.

Jennett, S. (1968) Assessment of respiratory effects of analgesic drugs. *British Journal of Anaesthesia* **40**: 746-756.

Jennett, S. (1976) Methods of studying the control of breathing in experimental animals and man. *Pharmacology and Therapeutics B.* **2.** 683-716.

Jennett, S., Barker, J. and Forrest, J.B. (1968) A double-blind controlled study of the effects on respiration of pentazocine, phenoperidine and morphine in normal man. *British Journal of Anaesthesia* **40**: 864-875

Orwin, J.M., Orwin, J., Price, M., (1976) A double-blind comparison of buprenorphine and morphine in conscious subjects following administration by the intramuscular route. *Acta Anaesthesiologica Belgica* **27** 171.

Read, D.J.C. (1967) A clinical method for assessing the ventilatory response to carbon dioxide. *Australasian Annals of Medicine* **16**: 20-32.

Smith, T.C., (1971) Pharmacology of respiratory depression. *International Anaesthesia Clinics.* **9** 125-143.

Weil, J.V., McCullough, R.E., Kline, J.S. & Sodal, I.E., (1975) Diminished ventilatory response to hypoxia and hypercapnia after morphine in normal man. *New England Journal of Medicine* **292** 1103-1106.

# 7. Cardiocirculatory effects of strong analgesic agents

A. D. MALCOLM AND D. J. COLTART

## Introduction

The experience of severe pain after surgery and trauma requires the therapeutic use of powerful analgesic agents. When the heart and circulation are normal the administration of doses of drugs sufficient to provide adequate analgesia is rarely precluded by unwanted haemodynamic effects. However, when the pain is of cardiac origin the clinical situation is more precarious and requires a knowledge of the haemodynamic action of the employed drug to ensure therapeutic safety. In this paper, particular emphasis will be placed on the treatment of pain in the early phase following acute myocardial infarction or following cardiac surgery with cardiopulmonary bypass.

There are five strong analgesic agents commonly in use in the United Kingdom, morphine, diamorphine, papaveretum, pethidine and pentazocine, and we shall deal first with these and conclude by mentioning some of our own work on buprenorphine, which we believe to be a promising new alternative to morphine.

It has been traditional to focus attention on those aspects of cardiocirculatory status most readily measured. Heart rate and arterial systolic, diastolic and mean pressure can readily be monitored in patients at the bedside or in the operating theatre and such observations therefore form the bulk of available data on effects in clinical use. However, in recent years interest has increased in the interrelationship between arterial pressure, blood flow and the effective hydraulic resistance or 'impedance' of the circulation (Greenfield, 1975; Milnor, 1975). For example, we illustrate in Figures 7.1 and 7.2 the effects of sodium nitroprusside, which relaxes peripheral arterioles and so reduces the effective hydraulic resistance of the peripheral circulation (Palmer and Lasseter, 1975). It is apparent that the nitroprusside infusion has profoundly reduced arterial systolic pressure from 158 mm Hg to 64 mm Hg but blood flow, measured by an electromagnetic transducer around the ascending aorta, has been maintained virtually unchanged (peak flow 11.61 litres/min. and 11.14 litres/min. respectively). Furthermore, measurement of left ventricular myocardial performance is a desirable element in the comprehensive evaluation of the circulatory effects of drugs but is difficult to achieve in clinical practice (Mirsky et al., 1974; Kolettis, Jenkins and Webb-Peploe, 1976; Mason et al., 1976) and data so far are scanty.

In the following sections we shall survey available data on the reviewed analgesic agents.

41

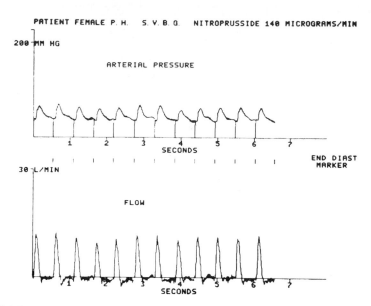

Fig. 7.1 Recording of arterial systolic pressure and blood flow in the ascending aorta before nitroprusside infusion.

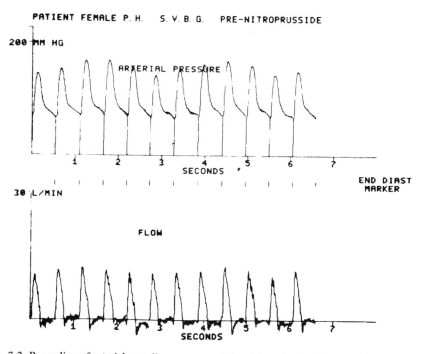

Fig. 7.2 Recording of arterial systolic pressure and blood flow during nitroprusside infusion.

## Morphine

This is considered first because it is so widely used and tends to be the yardstick against which other analgesic agents are judged. It has been known since the work of Drew, Dripps and Comroe (1946) that the effects of therapeutic doses are relatively unimportant in the supine normal subject, but hypotension and fainting are often seen with 75°head-up tilting or standing following intramuscular or intravenous injections of the drug. These effects are attributed largely to peripheral vasodilatation and are exacerbated in the presence of hypovolaemia. They are also exacerbated if phenothiazine drugs are administered concurrently (Jaffe and Martin, 1975, p.252). The opium alkaloids are histamine liberators, eliciting the triple response when injected in human skin, but this is probably not the sole mechanism of vasodilatation for there is also evidence of a depressor effect on the vasomotor centre (Reynolds and Randall, 1957, pp. 59-65). Rapid injection, large doses, and hypoxaemia accentuate the hypotensive effect, which may then become manifest even in the supine subject (Lowenstein et al., 1969; Wood-Smith, Vickers and Stewart, 1973, p. 192). When hypotension does occur, it can be reversed by postural adjustments, blood volume expansion or vasoactive agents (Lowenstein et al., 1969; Wood-Smith, Vickers and Stewart, 1973, p. 196). Larger doses of morphine slow the heart, chiefly by a central effect with some direct stimulation of the vagal nucleus (Reynolds and Randall, 1957, pp. 63 – 64).

In patients with acute myocardial infarction Thomas et al. (1965) gave intravenous morphine 3 to 10 mg with variable effect on heart rate, and blood pressure changes ranging from a small fall in pulse pressure to a large fall in arterial mean pressure. The hypotensive effect occurred soon after the intravenous injection and in one patient dramatic restoration of the arterial pressure was effected by raising the legs. In some patients whose blood pressure fell, cardiac output rose due to an increase in heart rate with or without an increase in stroke volume. Systemic vascular resistance remained unchanged in some patients and fell in others. The studies of Alderman et al. (1972) in patients with arteriographically proven coronary artery disease showed no consistent change in individual aortic pressures; the group mean value for aortic mean pressure was slightly, though not significantly, diminished. Pulmonary arterial mean pressure did not change. Whole-body oxygen consumption, cardiac index and left ventricular end-diastolic pressure all fell significantly after this 8 mg dose of intravenous morphine.

Morrison et al (1972) studied patients one hour after open heart surgery and measured heart rate, arterial and right atrial pressures, cardiac index and systemic vascular resistance. Morphine given intravenously in doses of 2.5 to 10.0 mg per 70 kilogram body weight caused no change in group mean values for any of the quantities. However, in individual patients both elevation and reduction in cardiac index were seen, unrelated to dose and with unpredictable alterations in arterial pressure. This variability is probably due to the different degrees of hypovolaemia, anaemia, hypoxaemia, catecholamine drive, electrolyte disturbance and myocardial dysfunction after cardiopulmonary bypass. In seven patients with aortic valve disease about to undergo aortic valve replacement (Lowenstein et al., 1969) enormous doses of morphine (0.5 to 1.0 mg per kilogram body weight) given intravenously resulted in significant increases in cardiac index, stroke index, central venous and pulmonary arterial pressures, and significant decrease in systemic vascular resistance. These changes were not seen in control subjects without cardiac disease who received 1.0 mg per kilogram body weight. The data of Lowenstein et al., (1969) in patients with chronically pressure or volume stressed hearts show no evidence of cardiac depression with these high doses of morphine. Experiments by Vasko et al., (1966a) on anaesthetised, open-chested dogs maintained on right heart bypass with crushed sino-atrial nodes and fixed-rate atrial pacing showed improved left ventricular function curves, improved myocardial contractile force and augmented left ventricular dp/dt with morphine 1.0 mg per kilogram body weight. However, when the dog experiments were extended to examine the effects of bilateral adrenalectomy or pharmacological beta adrenergic receptor blockade it appeared that the cardiostimulatory effects of morphine were indirect and the result of sympathoadrenal discharge. Pending definitive corroboration of this mechanism in man, caution should be exercised in administering morphine to beta blocked patients with cardiac dysfunction or to those with adrenal insufficiency.

Morphine is a traditional therapeutic agent in left ventricular failure and its mechanism of effect in this setting has been studied by Vasko et al. (1966b). Acute pulmonary oedema was provoked in dogs by producing mitral stenosis, aortic regurgitation, myocardial infarction or acute volume loading with saline given to animals with a previously constructed aortic coarctation. Morphine 0.5 mg per kilogram body weight resulted in the subsidence of pulmonary oedema in all animals and improvement was concomitant with striking and parallel decreases in pulmonary arterial pressure and flow and in left atrial and ventricular end-diastolic pressures. It seems that the principal mechanism of morphine's beneficial effect in pulmonary oedema is by increasing the capacity of the peripheral vascular bed and so producing a 'pharmacologic phlebotomy' (Vasko et al. 1966b).


### Diamorphine (Heroin)

The evidence of studies in various animal species suggests that the circulatory effects of diamorphine are similar to those of morphine (Reynolds and Randall, 1957, p.176). McDonald et al. (1967) studied the effects of a 5 mg intravenous dose of diamorphine in eight patients with acute myocardial infarction. Six patients were studied supine and aortic mean pressure, cardiac output, heart rate, stroke volume, systemic vascular resistance, pulmonary arterial pressure and right atrial pressure were measured. The only consistent and significant finding was a small fall in aortic mean pressure in the first 10 minutes after injection. In two additional patients 5 mg of diamorphine were administered intravenously with the patient tilted head-up at an angle of $10^{\circ}$ and there were no striking changes in any of the haemodynamic measurements in either patient, one of whom was markedly hypotensive. When the results of this study are compared with those of Thomas et al (1965) with 3 to 10 mg of intravenous morphine in the same clinical setting it appears that diamorphine is superior, for it provides adequate analgesia and sedation without unpleasant or harmful side effects and with less haemodynamic perturbation than morphine.


### Papaveretum (Omnopon)

This is a preparation of the water-soluble alkaloids of opium, standardised to contain

50 per cent anhydrous morphine. The remainder consists of hydrochlorides of other opiate alkaloids including papaverine, codeine, narcotine and thebaine (Wood-Smith *et al.*, 1973, pp. 198-200). Analgesic effects are principally due to the morphine content although there are additional beneficial effects from the other alkaloids, for papaverine reduces the tendency of morphine to cause nausea and vomiting, depression of respiration by morphine is less when papaverine is present, and narcotine potentiates the analgesic action of morphine. In the absence of information on haemodynamic effects with papaveretum, it can only be assumed that the effects of the morphine component predominate and in situations of compromised cardiovascular function the same precautions should be taken as with morphine.

## Pethidine (Meperidine)

Pethidine is structurally similar to atropine but there is no consistent effect on heart rate and its vagolytic effect is inconsequential (Reynolds and Randall, 1957, p.273 and p. 278; Wood-Smith *et al.*, 1973, pp. 200-202). It has a quinidine-like effect, reducing cardiac irritability (Wood-Smith *et al.*, 1973, p.202). Blood pressure is rarely affected by normal oral doses but with intravenous injection an abrupt, brief fall in pressure may be observed (Reynolds and Randall, 1957, pp. 276-278; Wood-Smith *et al.*, 1973, p. 202).

Rees *et al.* (1967) gave 100 mg of pethidine intravenously to eight patients with acute myocardial infarction and noted a biphasic response with an initial slight rise in arterial mean pressure, systemic vascular resistance and heart rate and then from 10 to 15 minutes a decline in these quantities to below control levels. Half of these patients experienced distressing dizziness and nausea. Rees *et al.*(1967) concluded that because of its circulatory effects, pethidine would not seem to be the ideal drug for the relief of pain in myocardial infarction. An initial increase in arterial mean pressure after pethidine has also been reported in healthy individuals (Prescott *et al.*, 1949) and in obstetric patients (Gallen and Prescott, 1944).

Pethidine is effective in the treatment of pulmonary oedema. Nadasdi and Zsoter (1969) gave intravenous pethidine 1 mg per kilogram body weight to 46 volunteers, six of whom had cardiac failure, and found that pethidine significantly increased blood flow in the forearm and leg with a concomitant fall in arterial and venous resistances. This is evidence that pethidine acts, like morphine, by promoting peripheral pooling of blood.

Tammisto *et al.* (1971) gave pethidine 2 mg per kilogram body weight intravenously to 10 patients with heart disease and found a brief rise in systolic blood pressure and then a fall to below control levels beyond 30 minutes. Heart rate showed a sustained elevation. Plasma adrenaline levels were unchanged and noradrenaline levels fell slightly. In additional experiments the effects of the same dose of intravenous pethidine on arterial blood pressure and heart rate response to exogenous catecholamines were assessed and it was found that the pressor responses to adrenaline and to noradrenaline were slightly augmented.

## Pentazocine

A dose of 20-30 mg has analgesic effect approximately equivalent to 10 mg of morphine (Wood-Smith *et al.*, 1973, p.200).

Pentazocine given intravenously in the rather high dose of 1.2 mg per kilogram body weight to patients without heart disease caused an increase in circulating adrenaline and noradrenaline levels which was paralleled by an increase in both blood pressure and heart rate (Tammisto *et al.*1971). There was slight augmentation of the pressor response to exogenous catecholamines, but less than with pethidine. Reports by Lal, Savidge and Chhabra (1969), Scott and Orr (1969) and Jewitt, Maurer and Hubner (1970) show that smaller doses of pentazocine augmented arterial pressure in more than 80 per cent of subjects and pulmonary arterial pressure was also augmented in the majority of such patients (Scott and Orr, 1969; Jewitt *et al.*, 1970). Fifteen patients studied by Jewitt *et al.*, (1970) just after acute myocardial infarction were given 30 or 60 mg of pentazocine intravenously and with only one exception, given 60 mg, the pulmonary arterial mean pressure had risen after 10 minutes. Aortic pressure rose, but remained elevated only with the 60 mg doses. Systemic vascular resistance rose after the 60 mg doses. Left ventricular minute work rose in all patients but this was significant only at 20 minutes after 60 mg.

Alderman *et al.*, (1972) studied the effects of 48 mg of intravenous pentazocine in nine patients with proven coronary disease and found the aortic mean pressure was augmented by 13 per cent, left ventricular end-diastolic pressure by 20 per cent, pulmonary arterial mean pressure by 36 per cent, pulmonary vascular resistance by 79 per cent and systemic vascular resistance by 11 per cent. Cardiac work was increased by 22 per cent with pentazocine in contrast to an 8 per cent decrease in similar patients who were given 8 mg of intravenous morphine. Because an increase in cardiac work and left ventricular afterload is generally held to be undesirable in the period immediately following acute myocardial infarction, morphine would appear to be a superior analgesic for most patients in this situation. However, where pre-existing hypotension complicates the situation and where there is reason to suspect that compensatory sympathetic activity is already maximal, pentazocine might be a preferable alternative — as argued by Alderman *et al.* (1972).

## Buprenorphine

Data provided by the manufacturer indicate that in general the cardiocirculatory effects are directionally similar to, though less marked than, those with morphine. Buprenorphine does not appear to cause histamine release. In the manufacturer's report of Phase 1 studies carried out by Simpson and Buckley at the London Hospital in lightly anaesthetised subjects, bradycardia and mild hypotension were noted, but on only three occasions in 21 sets of observations was the fall in blood pressure as great as 20 mm Hg. Studies by Devaux *et al.* (literature supplied by manufacturer) on buprenorphine used as a peroperative analgesic showed a dose-dependent response in certain cardiocirculatory measurements. At doses of 1.5 and 2.0 g per kilogram body weight no statistically significant effects were identified but at 3.0 and 4.0 $\mu$g per kilogram there were reductions in heart rate, cardiac output, arterial systolic and diastolic pressures, left ventricular work and oxygen consumption. There was no alteration in systemic vascular resistance. Rather different effects were reported by De Castro and Parmentier (literature supplied by manufacturer) when buprenorphine 0.8 mg was given intravenously at the end of analgesic anaesthesia. Some degree of cardiovascular stimulation was noted with increases in heart rate, arterial pressure, central venous pressure and right ventricular pressure. These effects were always transient.

At St Thomas's Hospital we are now able to make detailed measurements of cardiocirculatory status in human subjects soon after open-heart surgery. Cardiopulmonary bypass during such procedures is associated with myocardial damage (Archie and Kirklin, 1973) and thus patients studied under these circumstances would be expected to have impaired myocardial performance. We feel that this is a particularly useful situation in which to study a new analgesic agent for, as has been shown with morphine in the situation of acute myocardial infarction, it is in the patients with depressed cardiac reserve that undesirable haemodynamic effects may be apparent even when no such effects have been seen in other studies on patients with normal hearts.

A number of our patients undergoing open-heart surgery have an extractable electromagnetic blood flow probe (Williams *et al.*, 1972) in position around the ascending aorta during the first 48 hours after surgery. We record the phasic aortic blood flow signal together with the arterial pressure from a micromanometer on an arterial cannula, electrocardiogram and mean left atrial pressure. These data are processed 'off-line' on a Varian 620/L-100 digital computer with 24 K of core (Figs. 7.3 and 7.4). A number of haemodynamic measurements (Table 7.1) are calculated for each beat in seven-second samples of data and listed with the sample means in the output. Figures 7.5 to 7.8 and Table 7.2 illustrate our experience with the first patient to whom buprenorphine was given under these circumstances and we used a dose of 6 μg per kilogram body weight delivered as an intravenous bolus injection over 30 seconds. This initial study confirms the lack of cardiocirculatory disturbance with this dose of buprenorphine and the studies are continuing.

See following pages for Figures 7.3 to 7.8 and Tables 7.1 and 7.2.

## Acknowledgements

We thank Mr B.T. Williams, consultant cardiothoracic surgeon, and the staff of the Intensive Care Unit, St Thomas's Hospital for making it possible to conduct post-operative patient studies. Buprenorphine data were collected by Dr. B. Houston and Mr F. Rosenfeldt. Financial support was provided by Reckitt & Colman Pharmaceutical Division and by the Ernest Kleinwort Charitable Trust and the Cyril Kleinwort Charitable Settlement. The secretarial services of Fiona Baile and Diana Burley are gratefully acknowledged.

48

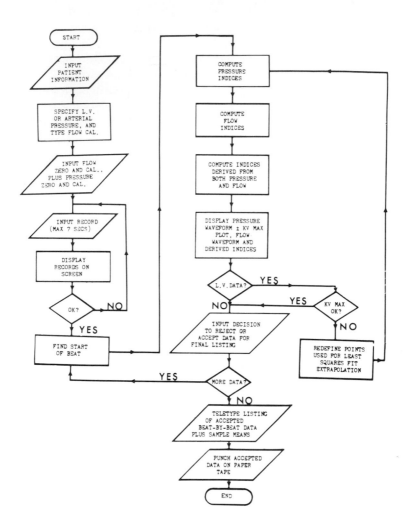

Fig. 7.3.

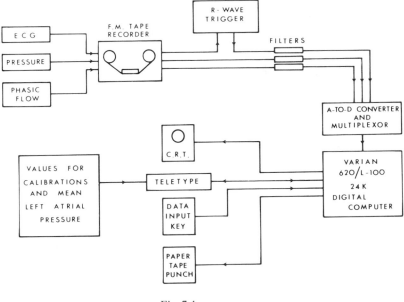

Fig. 7.4

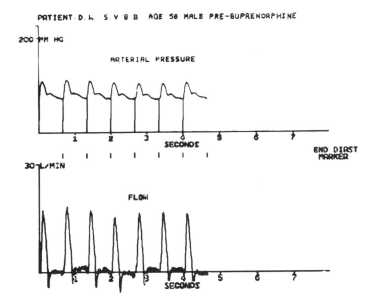

Fig. 7.5 Recording of arterial systolic pressure and blood flow in ascending aorta before buprenorphine injection.

Haemodynamic measurements computed and displayed beat – by – beat and listed with

sample means in final printout

| MEASUREMENT | ABBREVIATION | UNITS |
|---|---|---|
| R – R interval | R – R | secs |
| Aortic pressure, systolic | | mm Hg |
| Aortic pressure, diastolic | | mm Hg |
| Aortic pressure, mean | | mm Hg |
| Peak aortic blood flow | Max flow | litres $min^{-1}$ |
| Peak rate of change of aortic blood flow | Max dFlow/dt | litres $sec^{-2}$ |
| Stroke volume | | litres |
| 'Impedance' at maximum flow | Imp at max flow | $10^{-6}$ S.I. units of resistance |
| Mean systolic 'impedance' | Mean syst imp | $10^{-6}$ S.I. units of resistance |
| Stroke work | | joules |
| Peak left ventricular ejection power | Max L V ej power | watts |
| Mean left ventricular ejection power | Mean L V ej power | watts |
| Peak-rate-of change of ejection power | Max dPower/dt | watts $sec^{-1}$ |
| Percentage of forward aortic blood flow during first third | % flow to 33.3% syst | % |
| Ratio of diastolic pressure-time index to systolic tension-time index | DPTI/TTI | dimensionless |
| Duration of systole | syst | secs |

Table 7.1 Haemodynamic measurements computed and displayed beat-by-beat and listed with sample means in final printout.

50 year old man, saphenous vein bypass grafting,  buprenorphine 6 ug/kg

|  | 5 min | 10 min | 20 min |
|---|---|---|---|
| Heart rate | – 4% | – 8% | – 10% |
| Aortic pressure, systolic | – 1% | – 2% | + 1% |
| Aortic pressure, diastolic | – 1% | – 2% | – 1% |
| Aortic pressure, mean | – 1% | – 2% | – 1% |
| Peak flow | – 4% | – 8% | – 1% |
| Peak dFlow/dt | – 6% | – 8% | – 3% |
| Stroke volume | – 1% | – 5% | + 3% |
| 'Impedance' at maximum flow | + 3% | + 5% | + 2% |
| Mean systolic 'impedance' | + 1% | + 5% | + 2% |
| Stroke work | – 2% | – 6% | + 4% |
| Maximum ejection power | – 5% | –10% | – 2% |
| Maximum d Power/dt | – 8% | –11% | – 4% |
| Mean ejection power | – 4% | – 9% | – 1% |
| % flow in first ⅓ systole | 0% | + 3% | + 4% |
| DPTI/TTI | + 4% | +11% | + 7% |

Results are percentage changes from pre – buprenorphine control values

Table 7.2 Changes in haemodynamic measurements after intravenous injection of buprenorphine expressed as percentage changes from pre-injection control values.

52

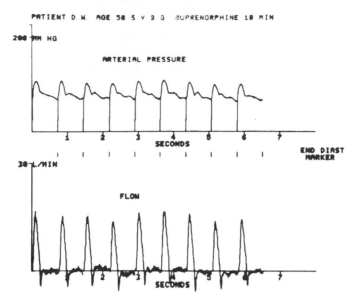

Fig. 7.6 Recording of arterial systolic pressure and blood flow in the ascending aorta 10 minutes after intravenous injection of buprenorphine.

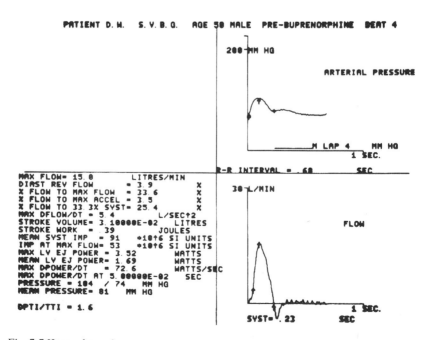

Fig. 7.7 Haemodynamic measurements before buprenorphine injection.

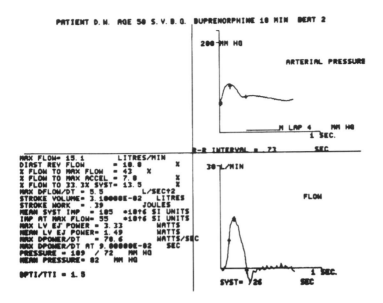

Fig. 7.8 Haemodynamic measurements 10 minutes after intravenous injection of buprenorphine.

## References

Alderman, E.L., Barry, W.H., Graham, A.F. and Harrison, D.C. (1972). Hemodynamic effects of morphine and pentazocine differ in cardiac patients. *New England Journal of Medicine,* **287,** 623-627.

Archie, J.P., Jr. and Kirklin, J.W. (1973). Myocardial blood flow and cardiac surgery. In *Advances in Cardiovascular Surgery* (J.W. Kirklin, ed.), pp. 189-203. New York: Grune and Stratton.

Drew, J.H., Dripps, R.D. and Comroe, J.H., Jr. (1946). Clinical studies on morphine. II. The effect of morphine upon the circulation of man and upon the circulatory and respiratory responses to tilting. *Anesthesiology,* 7, 44-61.

Gallen, B. and Prescott, F. (1944). Pethidine as an obstetric analgesic: a report on 150 cases. *British Medical Journal,* **1,** 176-179.

Greenfield, J.C., Jr. (1975). Methods and value of pulsatile blood flow measurements in man. In *Cardiovascular Clinics 6: 3 Diagnostic Methods in Cardiology* (N.O. Fowler, ed.), pp. 371-383. Philadelphia: F.A. Davis Co.

Jaffe, J.H. and Martin, W.R. (1975). Narcotic analgesics and antagonists. In *The Pharmacological Basis of Therapeutics,* fifth edition (L.S. Goodman and A. Gilman, eds.), pp. 245-283. New York: Macmillan.

Jewitt, D.E., Maurer, B.J. and Hubner, P.J.B. (1970). Increased pulmonary arterial pressures after pentazocine in myocardial infarction. *British Medical Journal,* **1,** 795-796.

Kolettis, M., Jenkins, B.S. and Webb-Peploe, M.M. (1976). Assessment of left ventricular function by indices derived from aortic flow velocity. *British Heart Journal,* **38,** 18-31.

Lal, S., Savidge, R.S. and Chhabra, G.P. (1969). Cardiovascular and respiratory effects of morphine and pentazocine in patients with myocardial infarction. *Lancet,* **1,** 379-381.

Lowenstein, E., Hallowell, P., Levine, F.H., Daggett, W.M., Austen, W.G and Laver, M.B. (1969). Cardiovascular response to large doses of intravenous morphine in man. *New England Journal of Medicine,* **281,** 1389-1393.

MacDonald, H.R., Rees, H.A., Muir, A.L., Lawrie, D.M., Burton, J.L. and Donald, K.W. (1967). Circulatory effects of heroin in patients with acute myocardial infarction. *Lancet,* **1,** 1070-1074.

Mason, D.T., Miller, R.R., Berman, D.S., Vismara, L.A., Williams, D.O., Salel, A.F., De Maria, A.N., Borgen, H.G., De Nardo, G.L. and Amsterdam, E.A. (1976). Cardiac catheterization in the clinical assessment of heart disease and ventricular performance. In *Congestive Heart Failure* (D.T. Mason, ed.), pp. 225-271. New York: Yorke Medical Books.

54

Milnor, W.R. (1975). Arterial impedance as ventricular afterload. *Circulation Research,* **36**, 565-57

Mirsky, I., Pasternac, A., Ellison, R.C. and Hugenholtz, P.G. (1974). Clinical applications of force-velocity parameters and the concept of a 'normalized velocity'. In *Cardiac Mechanics* (I. Mirsky, D.N. Ghista and H. Sandler, eds.), pp. 293-329. New York: John Wiley and Sons.

Morrison, J.D., Moffitt, E.A., Danielson, G.K. and Pluth, J.R. (1972). Circulatory effects of morphine early after open-heart surgery. *Journal of Thoracic and Cardiovascular Surgery,* **63**, 890-895.

Nadasdi, M. and Zsoter, T.T. (1969). The effect of meperidine on the peripheral circulation. *Clinical Pharmacology and Therapeutics,* **10**, 239-243.

Palmer, R.F. and Lasseter, K.C. (1975). Sodium nitroprusside. *New England Journal of Medicine,* **292**, 294-297.

Prescott, F., Ransom, S.G., Thorp, R.H. and Wilson, A. (1949). Effect of analgesics on respiratory response to carbon dioxide in man. *Lancet,* **1**, 340-344.

Rees, H.A., Muir, A.L., MacDonald, H.R., Lawrie, D.M., Burton, J.L. and Donald, K.W. (1967). Circulatory effects of pethidine in patients with acute myocardial infarction. *Lancet,* **2**, 863-866

Reynolds, A.K. and Randall, L.O. (1957). *Morphine and Allied Drugs.* Toronto: University of Toronto Press.

Scott, M.E. and Orr, R. (1969). Effects of diamorphine, methadone, morphine and pentazocine in patients with suspected acute myocardial infarction. *Lancet,* **1**, 1065-1067.

Tammisto, T., Jaattela, Nikki, P. and Takki, S. (1971). Effect of pentazocine and pethidine on plasma catecholamine levels. *Annals of Clinical Research,* **3**, 22-29.

Thomas, M., Malmcrona, R., Fillmore, S. and Shillingford, J. (1965). Haemodynamic effects of morphine in patients with acute myocardial infarction. *British Heart Journal,* **27**, 863-875.

Vasko, J.S., Henney, R.P., Brawley, T.K., Oldham, H.N. and Morrow, A.G. (1966 a). Effects of morphine on ventricular function and myocardial contractile force. *American Journal of Physiology,* **210**, 329-334.

Vasko, J.S., Henney, R.P., Oldham, H.N., Brawley, R.K. and Morrow, A.G. (1966 b). Mechanisms of action of morphine in the treatment of experimental pulmonary edema. *American Journal of Cardiology,* **18**, 876-883.

Williams, B.T., Sancho-Fornos, S., Clarke, D.B., Abrams, L.D., Shenk, W.G., Jr. and Barefoot, C.A. (1972). The Williams-Barefoot extractable blood flow probe – design, transducer characteristics and clinical applications in cardiac surgery. *Journal of Thoracic and Cardiovascular Surgery,* **63**, 917-921.

Wood-Smith, F.G., Vickers, M.D. and Stewart, H.C. (1973). *Drugs in Anaesthetic Practice,* 4th edition, London: Butterworths.

# Discussion

*Session 2*

*Dr Rosen.* In the study of the respiratory effects of analgesics which measurement is the most sensitive?

*Dr Jennett.* Current opinion is that some agreed index of the response to $CO_2$ is the best measure and at present it is accepted that displacement at say 20 litres per minute of ventilation would be acceptable. However, I am not convinced that this is any more reliable or repeatable than the actual increase in air breathing $PCO_2$.

*Dr James.* Does Dr Jennett consider that using the slope of the $CO_2$ response curve as an index of respiratory depression is satisfactory without indexing it to variation in $PO_2$?

*Dr Jennett.* In measurement of the response to $CO_2$ most authorities undertake such measurements at a high oxygen concentration.

One would expect that after a drug, as in the normal situation, the lower the $PO_2$ the greater would be the slope of the response to rising $CO_2$ unless peripheral chemoreceptors have been totally or partially blocked. Weil showed that there was a reduced response to hypoxia following morphine; if the chemoreceptor hypoxic drive is depressed by morphine one would not expect significant further depression by administration of oxygen.

Clinically, in the hypoxic patient receiving oxygen, depression is more likely with morphine than if it were withheld.

*Dr Dodson.* In such studies how can one be assured that psychological factors do not interfere with the results?

*Dr Jennett.* It is essential that the subjects are carefully prepared and are fully familiar with the apparatus and that the experiments are conducted in a quiet atmosphere with minimal disturbance. Under these conditions very consistent readings of air breathing $PCO_2$ can be recorded, and thus, while the increase following drug admini— stration is small, significant changes can be identified; in our studies changes in $CO_2$ response were less consistent although sometimes larger.

*Dr Houde.* How does sleep interfere with these measurements and how can you separate the drug effect from this?

*Dr Jennett.* Sleep will affect the measurement with a shift of the response; this effect cannot be separated from true drug effect and must be taken into account.

*Prof. Graham.* May I ask if the monitoring techniques used in ureteric colic are applicable to the biliary tract?

*Mr Watson.* This may be possible but is outside my sphere.

*Mr Rosenfeldt.* Although I am not aware of the results, techniques have been used at the Middlesex Hospital at the time of cholecystectomy to measure intra-biliary duct pressures and the effect of various flow rates down the duct under pressure to study resistance and the effects of drugs.

*Mr Rosenfeldt.* In studies of the cardiovascular effects of drugs with respiratory depressant effects, should the patient be allowed to breathe spontaneously, or should conditions be standardised by studying patients on ventilators with careful adjustment of blood gas levels?

*Dr James.* If you wish to accurately define a specific pharmacological effect, other conditions should be stabilised, whereas in the establishment of what will happen in clinical practice the effect on the whole organism should be studied. One must ask oneself is it a pharmacological or a clinical problem? It may well be both and you then have to do two experiments.

# Session 3    Chairman: J. D. P. Graham

# 8. Problems associated with strong analgesics

J. W. DUNDEE

## Introduction

As with any other type of drug, the problems associated with potent analgesics are not only the inherent effects of the drugs but also their modifications by the types of patients requiring such medication. However, analgesics are probably unique in that their side effects are different in type and severity in patients who require them and in normal pain-free, or anaesthetised subjects (Table 8.1). Furthermore, side

| Pain Sufferers | Pain Free |
| --- | --- |
| Euphoria: case of disconfort, worry and tension | Dysphoria: mild anxiety even fear |
| Nausea and vomiting in susceptible subjects | Frequent nausea and sickness |
| Depression antagonised by operative stimuli | Respiratory depression |
| Apathy and lethargy often desirable | Drowsiness undesirable |

Table 8.1 Side effects of analgesics in subjects with and without pain.

effects such as drowsiness are undesirable in the absence of pain but are often desirable in sufferers. Problems associated with analgesics should be viewed therefore in perspective. As an example, a small degree of respiratory depression may cause no problems in a patient with intractable pain of arthritic or neuritic origin, but may not be acceptable in a maternal analgesic, particularly in the presence of existing foetal distress.

## Classification of side effects

Bearing the above in mind, the side effects of potent analgesics can be considered in the same way as any other group of drugs and a workable classification of types of drug toxicity is shown in Table 8.2.

## TYPES OF DRUG TOXICITY

### Drug Action (Immediate)

a)   Inherent drug side effects

b)   Dose-related toxicity

c)   Hypersensitivity

d)   Local effects

e)   Interaction with other drugs

### Biotransformation Products (Delayed)

a)   Toxic effects

b)   Interaction with other drugs

Table 8.2 Classification of types of toxicity of potent analgesics.

## Biotransformation products

There is no evidence that the breakdown products or conjugated derivatives of clinical doses of potent analgesics cause delayed toxicity, even after prolonged use. The nearest approach to this is the simple cumulative action when relatively long acting drugs are given at frequent intervals; such a situation not infrequently arises when 10 mg methadone are given at four-hourly intervals after operation. Jaundice has been associated with prolonged parenteral use of analgesics but is likely to be the result of poor aseptic injection technique.

## Drug action (immediate)

Respiratory depression and nausea and/or vomiting are the most troublesome side effects of clinically used doses of potent analgesics. It has been assumed that there is an insuperable link between the analgesic potency of a compound and its respiratory depressant and emetic effects but the studies of Keats, Telford and Kurosu (1960) have thrown some doubt on this assumption. Further support for the concept of an opiate with minimal respiratory depressant action comes from studies with the effective respiratory stimulant, doxapram. Doses of 1.5 mg/kg which reverse the respiratory depressant action of morphine (20 mg/60 kg) do not affect the analgesic action of the opiate when given in the post operative period, nor reduce the efficacy of pethidine on experimentally-induced pain.(Gupta and Dundee, 1973, 1974, Gawley, Dundee and Jones, 1975). In contrast with doxapram, naloxone reverses both analgesia and respiratory depression; it is for this reason that the once popular preparation Pethilorfan (pethidine 100 mg, levallorphan 1.35 mg) is a less effective analgesic than pethidine alone. The anti-emetic, cyclizine, can be given with an opiate without any obvious antanalgesic action. Thus there is a definite possibility of an emetic-free analgesic with little respiratory depressant action.

Ample evidence exists to incriminate opiates as a cause of respiratory depression (Eckenhoff and Oech, 1960), although this may be hard to detect and its clinical importance is not always apparent. In fact measurements of respiratory rate and tidal volume, or even estimation of arterial $CO_2$ levels, may not always detect this effect; it may require sensitive techniques such as displacement of the $CO_2$ challenge curve to the right (Bellville and Fleischli, 1968). The respiratory depressant effects of potent analgesics only assume major clinical importance in normal patients during the post-operative period but must be kept in mind at all times in women at term and in patients with poor pulmonary function or cardiac disease.

Table 8.3 lists a number of factors which may influence the toxicity of potent

## FACTORS INFLUENCING THE TOXICITY OF

## POTENT ANALGESICS

Dosage

Route of administration

Rate of administration  (when given I.V.)

Movement  -  ambulation

Reason for use of drug  (± pain)

Previous or concurrent drug therapy

Individual susceptibility

Table 8.3 Factors influencing the toxicity of potent analgesics.

analgesics; the relative importance of these varies from patient to patient and also with different side effects. It has been suggested that there may be a biphasic emetic response to opiates with a decrease in the incidence of nausea and vomiting with very large doses. There is not universal agreement about this since Galway, Morrison and Dundee (1973) found a dose-related incidence of vomiting with doses up to 1.5 mg/kg pethidine and 0.2 mg/kg morphine with no constant increase thereafter. This also applies to the incidence of nausea with both of these commonly used drugs.

Patients who are prone to motion sickness are more likely to be sick after potent analgesics and both disturbance of the vestibular mechanism and stimulation of the chemoreceptor trigger zone can be incriminated as causative factors. Ambulant patients are more liable to sickness than those confined to bed and restriction of movement is a useful step in prevention of emesis.

Ambulation also increases the incidence of dizziness with opiates and this complication may be associated with minor degrees of postural hypotension. Morphine causes a significant decrease in systemic peripheral resistance and an increase in forearm blood flow (Samuel and Dundee, 1975). These two haemodynamic changes can explain all the cardiovascular effects of potent analgesics. The cardiovascular effects of these drugs are of little clinical importance except when they are given by rapid intravenous injection or to patients with cardiac disease or hypovolaemia.

The intravenous administration of analgesics during anaesthesia may result in a greater fall in blood pressure than in the awake patient. Vasodilators, such as promethazine, may also accentuate the depressant effects of opiates and in practice the combination of pethidine and diazepam is particularly liable to cause hypotension. There is some evidence to suggest that certain monoamine oxidase inhibitors may enhance the hypotensive effect of pethidine and similar drugs.

In Table 8.2 it will be noted that inherent drug side effects and drug related toxicity are listed separately. This indicates that not all side effects are dose related. As an example, some patients will not show emetic effects from any dose of a narcotic analgesic and yet some drugs are more likely to produce this effect than others. In contrast all clinically used analgesics show dose-related respiratory depression.

Psychotomimetic effects are a good example of a dose-related complication, but this is a common finding only in n-allyl opiates. This toxic manifestation places a limit on the upper acceptable dose of pentazocine, yet there is a marked individual susceptibility to this complication.

Muscular rigidity is another example of a side effect most frequently encountered with one group of drugs, as in clinical practice it occurs only with fentanyl and pethidine. Another group effect would seem to be the lesser constipating action of the piperidine compounds (pethidine, phenoperidine, fentanyl, anileridine) and greater effects of codeine derivatives as compared with other potent analgesics.

When the euphoriant and other side effects of potent analgesics are considered the circumstances under which they are used are of paramount importance (Table 8.1). Morphine causes euphoria and eases anxiety in the presence of pain while single doses may cause dysphoria, nausea and vomiting in normal subjects. Reference must be made to the addictive potential of potent analgesics, but a fuller discussion of this would be inappropriate here. It is sufficient to mention that those who, like Dr Cicely Saunders, frequently use diamorphine in hospices caring for the dying, do not find addiction to be a problem.

Some reference has already been made to the relative toxicity or lack of toxicity of individual drugs or groups of drugs. This has been discussed in many publications and only two studies, both from the author's department, will be discussed here. Dundee, Clarke and Loan (1965, 1967) compared the sedative-toxic effects of intramuscular doses of 100 mg pethidine and 10 mg morphine over a four hour period. The differences could all be explained on the basis of the rate of onset and relative duration of action of these popular drugs. Pethidine has an earlier onset of action than morphine and this accounts for the higher incidence of 'early' vomiting when it is given as preanaesthetic medication. In contrast, the slower and longer acting morphine causes delayed, but prolonged, vomiting. In later studies, it was noted that the time course of action of diamorphine resembled that of pethidine while methadone resembled morphine in this respect.

As a result of a major study of many opiates given in their usual adult clinical doses for preanaesthetic medication, Dundee, Loan and Morrison (1970) classed their incidence of emetic symptoms as being less or more than average for the pooled total involving all the drugs (Table 8.4). Table 8.5 shows a similar grading of overall

| | | | |
|---|---|---|---|
| SIGNIFICANTLY LESS | Dipipanone | 1.5 | mg |
| | Dihydrocodeine | 50 | mg |
| LESS | Phenazocine | 2 | mg |
| | Dextromoramide | 5 | mg |
| | Pentazocine | 30 | mg |
| | Phenoperidine | 2 | mg |
| AVERAGE | ANILERIDINE | 45 | mg |
| | DIAMORPHINE | 5 | mg |
| | METHADONE | 10 | mg |
| | PETHIDINE | 100 | mg |
| MORE | Fentanyl | 0.2 | mg |
| | Levorphanol | 2 | mg |
| | Oxycodone | 10 | mg |
| | Morphine | 10 | mg |
| SIGNIFICANTLY MORE | Oxymorphone | 1.5 | mg |
| | Dihydromorphinone | 2 | mg |
| | Papaveretum | 20 | mg |

Drugs are placed in rank order of toxicity, as described by Dundee, Loan and Morrison (1970).

Table 8.4 Relative incidence of emetic effects of potent analgesics when given I.M. for preanaesthetic medication to adult women of reproductive years.

| | | | |
|---|---|---|---|
| SIGNIFICANTLY LESS | Phenazocine | 2 | mg |
| | Dihydrocodeine | 50 | mg |
| LESS | Phenoperidine | 2 | mg |
| | Dipipanone | 25 | mg |
| | Methadone | 10 | mg |
| | Dextromoramide | 5 | mg |
| | Oxycodone | 10 | mg |
| | Anileridine | 45 | mg |
| | Levorphanol | 2 | mg |
| AVERAGE | MORPHINE | 10 | mg |
| | DIAMORPHINE | 5 | mg |
| MORE | Fentanyl | 0.2 | mg |
| | Pentazocine | 30 | mg |
| | Papaveretum | 20 | mg |
| SIGNIFICANTLY MORE | Dihydromorphinone | 2 | mg |
| | Oxymorphone | 1.5 | mg |
| | Pethidine | 100 | mg |

Drugs are placed in rank order of toxicity, as described by Dundee, Loan and Morrison (1970)

Table 8.5 Relative overall toxicity of usual doses of potent analgesics when given I.M. for preanaesthetic medication to adult women of reproductive years.

62

incidence and severity of side effects. The median position of morphine in both of these comparisons is very obvious but there were no major differences in the relative toxicity of the currently available analgesics.

References

Bellville, J.W. and Fleischli, G. (1968). The interaction of morphine and nalorphine on respiration. *Clinical Pharmacology and Therapeutics,* 9, 152-161.

Dundee, J.W., Clarke, R.S.J. and Loan, W.B. (1965). Comparison of the sedative and toxic effects of morphine and pethidine. *Lancet,* 2, 1262-1263.

Dundee, J.W., Clarke, R.S.J. and Loan, W.B. (1967). Comparative toxicity of diamorphine, morphine and methadone. *Lancet,* 1, 221-223.

Dundee, J.W., Loan, W.B., Morrison, J.D. (1970). Studies of drugs given before anaesthesia XIX. The opiates. *British Journal of Anaesthesia,* 42, 54-58.

Eckenhoff, J.E. and Oech, S.R. (1960). The effects of narcotics and antagonists upon respiration and circulation in man. A review. *Clinical Pharmacology and Therapeutics,* 1, 483-524.

Galway, J.E., Morrison, J.D. and Dundee, J.W. (1973). Dosage/side-effect relationships of morphine and meperidine. *Anesthesia and Analgesia...Current Researches,* 52, 536-541.

Gawley, T.H., Dundee, J.W. and Jones, C.J. (1975). The role of doxapram in the reduction of pulmonary complications following surgery. *British Journal of Anaesthesia,* 47, 906-907.

Gupta, P.K. and Dundee, J.W. (1973). Alterations in response to somatic pain associated with anaesthesia XXII: Nikethamide, doxapram and naloxone. *British Journal of Anaesthesia,* 45, 497-500.

Gupta, P.K. and Dundee, J.W. (1974). Morphine combined with doxapram or naloxone. A study of postoperative pain relief. *Anaesthesia,* 29, 33-39.

Keats, A.S., Telford, J. and Kurosu, Y. (1960). Studies of analgesic drugs IV. Dissociation of analgesic, respiratory and emetic effects. *Journal of Pharmacology,* 130, 218-221.

Samuel, I.O. and Dundee, J.W. (1975). Circulatory effects of morphine. *British Journal of Anaesthesia,* 47, 1025-1026.

# 9. Pharmacological advances in analgesics

H. W. KOSTERLITZ

Our knowledge of the mode of action of narcotic analgesics is still fragmentary. We
really do not know how they act at a cellular and molecular level. If one wants to
make progress in this direction, the foremost task is the identification of suitable
and relatively simple models, because  the central nervous system has such a heterogeneous
structure that it would be impossible to separate the morphine-sensitive neurones
from those which do not respond to morphine. As a result of work in the last 10 years,
we now have a number of models which we can use for an investigation of this
problem. Two of these models are of a pharmacological character. The first one is
based on the fact that, in the guinea-pig ileum, impulse transmission from the myenteric
plexus to the smooth muscle is depressed by very low concentrations of morphine. A
second model with similar pharmacological properties is the mouse *vas deferens*. A
different type of model depends on the binding of opiates and opioid peptides to
membrane fragments of nerve terminals in the central and peripheral nervous systems,
a field pioneered by A. Goldstein, E.J. Simon, L. Terenius and S.H. Snyder. In the
fourth model, cultured cells of a hybrid neuroblastoma x glioma clone are used, in
which all characteristics of the pharmacological action of opiates, including tolerance
and dependence, can be demonstrated. What I want to do now is to discuss briefly
some aspects of these models and then to say something about the most recent
results stemming from these investigations, namely the discovery of the endogenous
opioid peptides.

Figure 9.1. shows that there is a close correlation between the potencies of
narcotic analgesics to depress the electrically induced contractions of the guinea-pig
ileum and the clinical data on analgesia in man (Kosterlitz and Waterfield, 1975).
The solid line is the theoretical line for perfect correlation, while the interrupted line
is the regression line calculated from the data. Although the potencies of the compounds
vary over five orders of magnitude, the correlation is surprisingly good, particularly
when you consider that we are dealing with two different species and have to take
into account the difficulties encountered in the quantitative assessment of analgesia
in man; in addition, there are the problems of absorption and bio-transformation
affecting the human data. This close correlation was the first indication that the
guinea-pig ileum was likely to be suitable for an investigation into the mode of action
of narcotic analgesics.

Figure 9.2. shows the results obtained on the second, more recent model, the
mouse *vas deferens;* the relative agonist potencies in the mouse *vas deferens* have

64

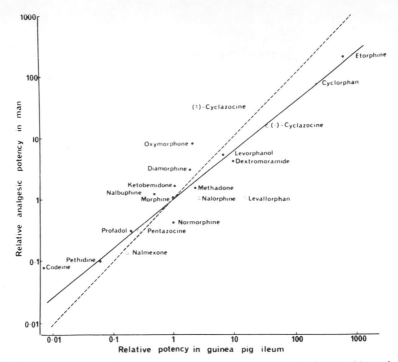

Fig. 9.1. Correlation between the relative agonist potencies in guinea-pig ileum and in analgesia in man (morphine = 1). The effects in segments of guinea-pig ileum are measured by the depression of the isometric contractions of the longitudinal muscle evoked by coaxial stimulation (0.1 Hz, 0.5 ms, supramaximal voltage). Reproduced with permission from Kosterlitz and Waterfield (1975), *Annual Review of Pharmacology,* **15.** Copyright © 1975 by Annual Reviews Inc. All rights reserved.

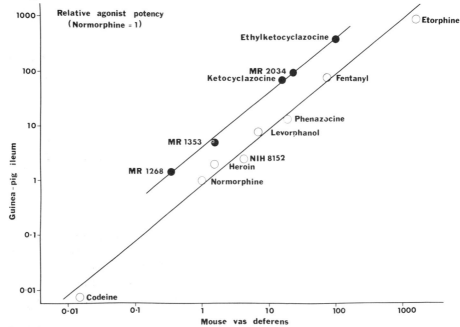

Fig. 9.2. Relative agonist activities of various narcotic analgesic agonists in the mouse *vas deferens* and guinea-pig ileum (normorphine = 1). The compounds fitting the regression line on the right substitute and those fitting the line on the left (benzomorphans) do not substitute for morphine in the morphine-dependent monkey. Reproduced from Lord, Waterfield, Hughes and Kosterlitz (1977), with permission from *Nature,* **267,** Macmillan Journals Ltd.

been correlated with those in the guinea-pig ileum (Hughes, Kosterlitz and Leslie, 1975). The line on the right shows that a large number of narcotic analgesics fall on a straight line with a slope of near unity, indicative of a good correlation between the two sets of data. A second line has been drawn to the left of the first one; we have here a number of compounds which are all benzomorphans and related to cyclazocine. Ketocyclazocine and ethylketocyclazocine are Sterling Winthrop compounds, while the Mr-compounds were obtained from C.H. Boehringer, Ingelheim. They have one thing in common, namely that they are good antinociceptive agents which, however, will not substitute for morphine in the morphine-dependent monkey. We do not know yet whether these compounds can be used in human clinical work. What is of interest is the fact that in our two models they behave differently from the classical narcotic analgesics. First, they are all much less potent in the mouse *vas deferens* than in the guinea-pig ileum and, secondly, they require more naloxone for antagonism than the classical opiates. We concluded from these findings that the receptor populations in the guinea-pig ileum and the mouse *vas deferens* are not identical and are probably heterogeneous (Hutchinson *et al*, 1975).

In other words, and I cannot give the whole evidence, we have more than one opiate receptor. This was our first indication that the opiate receptor system may be very complex, a concept to which I shall return during the discussion of the endogenous opioid peptides.

Lipid solubility influences the action of narcotic analgesics. The next figure (Fig. 9.3.) shows the rates of onset and offset of the actions of normorphine and levorphanol in the guinea-pig ileum. Both the onset and offset of the effect of normorphine are rapid whereas the onset and offset of action of levorphanol are much slower. We thought that these differences might possibly be due to differences in lipid solubility, since normorphine is much less lipid soluble than levorphanol.

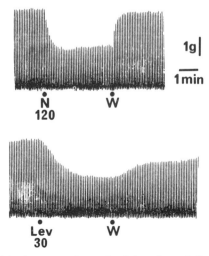

Fig. 9.3. Contractions of the longitudinal muscle of the guinea-pig ileum evoked by electrical field stimulation (0.2 Hz, 1 ms, supramaximal voltage). Upper tracing: at N, normorphine added (120 nM) and at W, washed out. Lower tracing: at Lev, levorphanol added (30 nM) and at W, washed out. Reproduced from Kosterlitz, Leslie and Waterfield (1975), with permission from European Journal of Pharmacology, 32, Elsevier/North Holland, Biomedical Press, Amsterdam.

Table 9.1. gives a number of compounds with very different lipid solubilities (Kosterlitz, Leslie and Waterfield, 1975). Normorphine has the lowest and buprenorphin the highest lipid solubility, levorphanol and etorphine being intermediary. The table shows that in the guinea-pig ileum, the relative agonist potency is not correlated with lipid solubility. On the other hand, there is a strong correlation between the half-times of onset and lipid solubility: the more hydrophilic a compound is, the more rapid are its onset and offset of action, and the more lipid soluble it is, the slower are the onset and offset. Obviously this is a very important phenomenon. It is quite different from what we would expect from observations in *in vivo* experiments, where lipid solubility facilitates passage through the blood brain barrier. Thus, lipid solubility acts in two opposing directions: *in vitro,* where we measure mainly receptor properties, high lipid solubility will favour slow onset and long duration of action, whereas *in vivo* the same properties will ensure a rapid onset of action and by rapid removal of the drug from the brain shorten the duration of action.

| Drug | Relative agonist potency | Half-times (s) of Onset | Offset |
|---|---|---|---|
| Normorphine | 1 | 11 | 22 |
| Morphine | 1 | 23 | 32 |
| Levorphanol | 7.5 | 75 | 268 |
| Etorphine | 700 | 74 | 211 |
| Methadone | 3 | 91 | 619 |
| Buprenorphine | 220 | 623 | very long |

The drugs have been arranged in ascending order of lipid solubility.

Table 9.1. The effect of lipid solubility on the rates of onset and offset of action in the guinea-pig ileum.

What is even more important is the interaction between the agonists and antagonists. The interaction between the agonist methadone, which is highly lipid soluble, and the quaternary antagonist N-methylnalorphinium which has a low lipid solubility and therefore a very rapid onset of action with a short duration is shown in Figure 9.4. Methadone was added first. As expected, the onset of action was slow; when equilibrium had been reached, the addition of the antagonist caused a very rapid reversal of the depressant effect of methadone. Then both agonist and antagonist were washed out and, since the duration of action of methadone is longer than that of the antagonist, the depression of the contraction recurred. This observation is of obvious clinical importance in circumstances when a short-acting antagonist is used to reverse the effect of a long-acting agonist.

We shall now discuss some of the results obtained with the cultured neuroblastoma x glioma cells. This work was initiated by Nirenberg and Klee at the National Institute

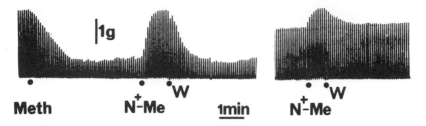

**Meth**          **N⁺-Me**    **W**    **1min**    **N⁺-Me**    **W**

Fig. 9.4. Contractions of the longitudinal muscle of the guinea-pig ileum. Effect of the quaternary antagonist, N-methylnalorphinium (N ± Me, 600 nM) on the rate of recovery from the depressant action of methadone (Meth, 260 nM). No methadone was added to the bath after the first wash-out, W. Between the two tracings there was an interval of 14 min. From Kosterlitz, Leslie and Waterfield (1975), with permission, European Journal of Pharmacology, **32**, Elsevier/North Holland, Biomedical Press, Amsterdam.

of Mental Health. In Figure 9.5. there are two regression lines for each drug. The interrupted line shows the inhibition of [³H]naloxone binding by the drug while the solid line indicates the effect on the cyclic AMP content of an homogenate of the cells (Sharma, Nirenberg and Klee, 1975). Agonists, such as morphine, etorphine and levorphanol, inhibit [³H]-naloxone binding and depress the action of adenylate cyclase. On the other hand, the antagonist naloxone inhibits binding but has no effect on the activity of adenylate cyclase. It is well known that dextrophan, the dextro-isomer of the potent analgesic levorphanol, has no analgesic properties and it is therefore interesting that dextrophan does not inhibit adenylate cyclase and decreases [³H] -naloxone binding only in concentrations very much higher than those at which levorphanol is effective. Thus, stereospecificity of narcotic analgesics can be demonstrated on this model.

These authors have also shown (Sharma, Klee and Nirenberg, 1975) that the cultured neuroblastoma x glioma hybrid cells become tolerant to the action of opiates and that after their withdrawal, there is an increase in the activity of adenylate cyclase, a phenomenon which may be related to the syndrome of withdrawal observed in the whole animal.

Let us now consider the endogenous opioid peptides. The formula of methionine-enkephalin is shown in Figure 9.6. It consists of five amino acids: tyrosine, glycine, glycine, phenylalanine and methionine. (Hughes, *et al.,* 1975). When methionine is replaced by leucine, we obtain the second pentapeptide found in brain, leucine-enkephalin.

I shall now explain one of the most exciting events in the whole history of enkephalins, namely the discovery that methionine-enkephalin is present as amino acid sequence 61-65 in a large peptide consisting of 91 amino acid residues, *Beta*-lipotropin which was first isolated from the pituitary by Li, Barnafi, Chrétien and Chung (1965) (Fig. 9.7). It is of interest that all peptides starting with tyrosine at position 65 have analgesic activity. This effect is transient with the short peptide, methionine-enkephalin, because it is very easily inactivated by peptidases in the brain. On the other hand, the peptides consisting of 16 amino acids or more are resistant to the action of these enzymes and of these peptides, C-fragment or *Beta*-endorphin (61-91) is the most potent analgesic with a long duration of action (Bradbury *et al,* 1976).

68

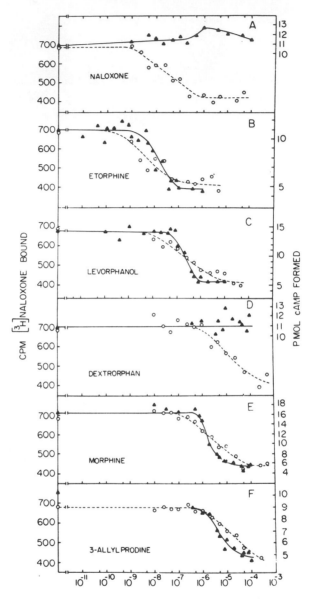

Fig. 9.5. The effectiveness of various narcotics as inhibitors of adenylate cyclase activity of NG108–15 homogenates is compared with their ability to displace [³H]-naloxone (o) bound to receptor: [³²P]-cAMP formed per min per tube (250μg of protein per tube). Reproduced from Sharma, Nirenberg and Klee (1975).

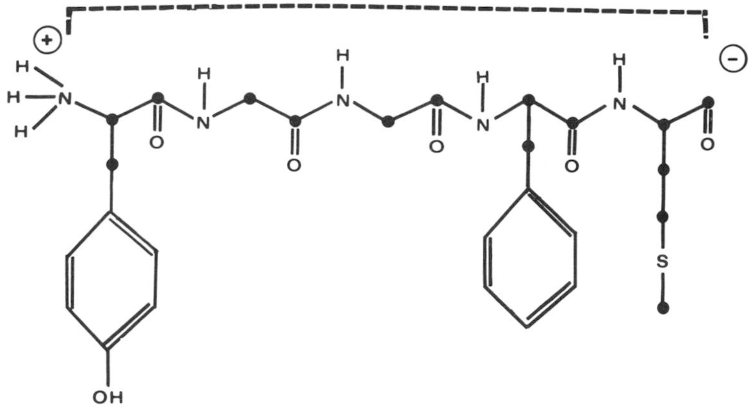

Fig. 9.6. Formula of methionine-enkephalin. Reproduced from Kosterlitz and Hughes (1977), with permission from British Journal of Psychiatry, **130**.

H-Glu-Leu-Thr-Gly-Gln-Arg-Leu-Arg-Gln-Gly- <sup>10</sup>

Asp-Gly-Pro-Asn-Ala-Gly-Ala-Asn-Asp-Gly- <sup>20</sup>

Glu-Gly-Pro-Asn-Ala-Leu-Glu-His-Ser-Leu- <sup>30</sup>

Leu-Ala-Asp-Leu-Val-Ala-Ala-Glu-Lys-Lys- <sup>40</sup>

Asp-Glu-Gly-Pro-Tyr-Arg-Met-Glu-His--Phe- <sup>50</sup>

Arg-Trp-Gly-Ser-Pro-Pro-Lys-Asp-Lys-Arg- <sup>60</sup>

Tyr-Gly-Gly-Phe-Met-Thr-Ser-Glu-Lys-Ser- <sup>70</sup>

Gln-Thr-Pro-Leu-Val-Thr-Leu-Phe-Lys-Asn- <sup>80</sup>

Ala-Ile-Ile-Lys-Asn-Ala-Tyr-Lys-Lys-Gly- <sup>90</sup>

Glu-OH.

Fig. 9.7. Amino acid sequence of human *Beta*-lipotropin as determined by Li and Chung (1976).

As far as distribution is concerned, enkephalin and leucine-enkephalin are unevenly distributed in the brain and present in high concentrations in those areas in which neurones mediating the pain pathway are found, as for instance, the substantia gelatinosa and the periventricular grey. On the other hand, C-fragment or *Beta*-endorphin is present in very high concentrations in the intermediate and anterior lobes of the pituitary (Bradbury *et al.*, 1976; Bloom *et al*, 1977) and, in much lower concentrations, also in the brain.

I should now like to return to the hypothesis that there is more than one opiate receptor. We have tested the enkephalins, *Beta*-endorphin and its fragments of various lengths on the contractions of the guinea-pig ileum and the mouse *vas deferens* and on the inhibition of [3H]-naloxone and [3H]-leucine-enkephalin binding in brain homogenates. We have arrived at the conclusion that the results cannot be explained on the basis of a single opiate receptor and postulate that there are at least two and probably more species of receptors. *Beta*-endorphin interacts equally well with both receptors whereas the enkephalins interact much better with the receptor which has a higher affinity for the [$^3$H]-leucine-enkephalin binding site than for the [$^3$H]-naloxone binding site. In contrast, morphine has a higher affinity for the [$^3$H]-naloxone binding site than for the [$^3$H]-leucine-enkephalin binding site. The experimental evidence is presented by Lord *et al* (1977).

I want to end this paper with one or two speculations which may be of some interest. I have already mentioned that *Beta*-endorphin, the long peptide, is present in the pituitary in high concentrations. We do not know yet whether it is released from the pituitary into the blood stream, but after intravenous injection it passes through the blood brain barrier and exerts its analgesic action. It has been found that it stimulates prolactin release and may possibly be involved in the control of the release of other pituitary hormones. Its onset of action is considerably slower than that of the enkephalins and it has a much longer duration of action. It would appear then that *Beta*-endorphin may have a neurohumoral function in contrast to the enkephalins which have a rapid onset of action which is of short duration due to inactivation by peptidases. The enkephalins would therefore appear to be more suitable as neurotransmitters or neuromodulators (Hughes and Kosterlitz, 1977; Kosterlitz and Hughes, 1977). In view of the very high concentrations of *Alpha*-endorphin (61–76) and particularly *Beta*-endorphin (61–91) in the anterior and intermediate lobes of the pituitary, we wonder whether it could be possible that these endorphins are involved in the fight and flight reaction in a manner similar to the role played by the adrenaline present in the adrenal medulla. It is an old-established fact that soldiers on the battlefield do not notice when they are severely injured. This insensitivity to severe pain may possibly be due to secretion of endorphins. Is it likely that women in childbirth have an increased secretion of these endorphins?

### References

Bloom, F., Battenberg, E., Rossier, J., Ling, N., Leppaluoto, J., Vargo, T.M. and Guillemin, R. (1977). Endorphins are located in the intermediate and anterior lobes of the pituitary gland, not in the neurohypophysis. *Life Sciences,* **20,** 43–48.

Bradbury, A.F., Feldberg, W.F., Smyth, D.G. and Snell, C.R. (1976). Lipotropin C-fragment: an endogenous peptide with potent analgesic activity. In *Opiates and Endogenous Opioid Peptides,* pp. 9–17. Amsterdam, North-Holland Publishing Co.

Hughes, J. and Kosterlitz, H.W. (1977). Opioid peptides. *British Medical Bulletin,* **33,** 157–161.

Hughes, J., Kosterlitz, H.W. and Leslie, F.M. (1975). Effect of morphine on adrenergic transmission in the mouse *vas deferens.* Assessment of agonist and antagonist potencies of narcotic analgesics. *British Journal of Pharmacology,* **53,** 371–381.

Hughes, J., Smith, T.W., Kosterlitz, H.W., Fothergill, L.A., Morgan, B.A. and Morris, H.R. (1975). Identification of two related pentapeptides from the brain with potent opiate agonist activity. *Nature,* **258,** 577–579.

Hutchinson, M., Kosterlitz, H.W., Leslie, F.M., Waterfield, A.A. and Terenius, L. (1975). Assessment in the guinea-pig ileum and mouse *vas deferens* of benzomorphans which have strong antinociceptive activity but do not substitute for morphine in the dependent monkey. *British Journal of Pharmacology,* **55,** 541–546.

Kosterlitz, H.W. and Hughes, J. (1977). Peptides with morphine-like action in the brain. *British Journal of Psychiatry,* **130,** 298–304.

Kosterlitz, H.W., Hughes, J., Lord, J.A.H. and Waterfield, A.A. (1977) Enkephalins, endorphins and opiate receptors. *Neuroscience Symposia,* **2,** in press.

Kosterlitz, H.W., Leslie, F.M. and Waterfield, A.A. (1975). Rates of onset and offset of action of narcotic analgesics in isolated preparations. *European Journal of Pharmacology,* **32,** 10–16.

Kosterlitz, H.W. and Waterfield, A.A. (1975). *In vitro* models in the study of structure-activity relationships of narcotic analgesics. *Annual Reviews of Pharmacology,* **15,** 29–47.

Li, C.H., Barnafi, L., Chrétien, M. and Chung, D. (1965). Isolation and amino-acid sequences of *Beta*-LPH from sheep pituitary glands. *Nature,* **208,** 1093−1094.

Li, C.H. and Chung, D. (1976). Primary structure of human *Beta*-lipotropin. *Nature,* **260,** 622−624.

Lord, J.A.H., Waterfield, A.A., Hughes, J. and Kosterlitz, H.W. (1977). Endogenous opioid peptides : multiple agonists and receptors. *Nature,* **267,** 495−499.

Sharma, S.K., Klee, W.A. and Nirenberg, M. (1975). Dual regulation of adenylate cyclase accounts for narcotic dependence and tolerance. *Proceedings of the National Academy of Sciences, U.S.A.,* **72,** 3092−3096.

Sharma, S.K., Nirenberg, M. and Klee, W.A. (1975). Morphine receptors as regulators of adenylate cyclase activity. *Proceedings of the National Academy of Sciences, U.S.A.,* **72,** 590−594.

## Discussion

*Session 3*

*Dr Houde.* Could Prof. Kosterlitz explain how Dr Terenius's report showing elevated levels of morphine-like factors in cerebrospinal fluid correlates with his concept of how these may be functioning in the central nervous system?

*Prof. Kosterlitz.* This is difficult; Dr Terenius and his colleagues found two chromatographically different peptides in human c.s.f. One (fraction II) is probably identical with enkephalin, the other (fraction I) is not. He found that in severe pain there was a decrease in fraction I but not in fraction II. However, at present, these observations cannot be related to any of the concepts I discussed.

*Dr Rosen.* Why does naloxone not cause pain in man by antagonising endorphins?

*Prof. Kosterlitz.* This is a very important point which has concerned many people working in this field (cf. El-Sobky, Dostrovsky and Wall, 1976). There is, however, evidence that naloxone can alter the pain threshold. For instance, it has been shown that electro-acupuncture raises the pain threshold to electrical stimulation of a tooth in man and that this phenomenon is reversed by injection of naloxone but not of saline (Mayer, Price and Rafii, 1977). It has also been shown that in rats, naloxone causes an increase in the nociceptive responses to thermal stimuli and that in dogs it leads to mydriasis, tachypnoea, tachycardia, agitation and hyperthermia (Jacob, Tremblay and Colombel, 1974; Jacob and Michaud, 1976).

May I use this opportunity to raise the question of side effects of opiates? If the opioid peptides have a physiological function, then it may be assumed that at least some of the so-called side effects are exaggerated physiological functions of the peptidergic system. For instance, there is a high density of opiate receptors and also a high concentration of enkephalins in the striatum; two of the side effects we can readily demonstrate in rodents after administration of opiates and endorphins are catatonia and catalepsy. Furthermore, the depression of respiration seen after opiates and opioid peptides may be only the exaggerated response to compounds involved in the physiological control of respiration.

*Prof. Joslin.* Following Prof. Kosterlitz's comments on the long peptides and the pituitary I would like to report a clinical observation in this regard. It is well recognised that in advanced breast cancer pituitary ablation is followed by relief of pain. Using radioactive yttrium a large percentage of patients experience pain relief within 24 hours which is unrelated to other therapy. Could he comment on whether this is stimulation of the encephalon or is it post-operative pituitary stimulation, as I presume this is where the long peptides originate?

*Prof. Kosterlitz.* It is impossible to answer your question because at present we have no satisfactory radio-immunoassay for the long-chain endorphins. Candace Pert and her colleagues (Pert, Pert and Tallman, 1976) have published a paper in which they describe a compound, anodynin, which they obtained from human plasma and which interacts with the opiate receptor. This substance may be relevant to the question you raised.

As long as we are unable to determine the endorphins directly, it may be of interest to study their possible effects on hormones released from the pituitary. They are known to cause release of prolactin; it is possible that they may reduce LH and testosterone levels in serum. Have you tested for this?

*Prof. Joslin.* No, we have not checked but this is something occurring within 24 hours. If we induce LH changes by other means we do not necessarily get pain relief.

*Prof. Kosterlitz.* It was shown recently in rats by Cicero and his colleagues (Cicero *et al.* 1976) that a single injection of morphine reduced the serum LH level by 50 per cent or more in one hour and the testosterone level by more than 80 per cent in three to four hours.

*Prof. Graham.* I have recently visited Hong Kong to study problems of narcotic dependence. In dealing with large numbers of such patients cost effectiveness is most important and if withdrawal can be achieved quickly this would save much time and effort. This can be produced with naloxone but this creates its own problems. A method which I saw demonstrated consisted of electrical acupuncture to the ear which creates a buzz. Naloxone is then administered for three consecutive days and no acute withdrawal is produced.

Can Prof. Kosterlitz correlate this with release of endorphins and if so how does this relate to naloxone producing its effect but not being appreciated?

*Prof. Kosterlitz.* This observation is difficult to interpret.

*Dr Geddes.* I think there is something higher up than the pituitary controlling these mechanisms.

*Prof. Kosterlitz.* While so far nothing is known about the mechanisms for the release of endorphins, it is possible that the hypothalamus plays an important role.

*Dr Burn.* It has been observed that the use of regional blockade in patients controlled on large doses of narcotic analgesics who then cease taking the narcotic, is not followed by withdrawal symptoms. Can Prof. Kosterlitz explain this?

*Prof. Kosterlitz.* This is an interesting observation but cannot be explained in our present state of knowledge.

### References

Cicero, T.J., Wilcox, C.E., Bell, R.D. and Meyer, E.R. (1976) Acute reductions in serum testosteron levels by narcotics in the male rat: stereospecificity, blockade by naloxone and tolerance. *Journal of Pharmacology and Experimental Therapeutics, 198*, 34–346.

El–Sobky, A., Dostrovsky, J.O. and Wall, P.D. (1976). Lack of effect of naloxone on pain perception in humans. *Nature, 263*, 783–784.

Jacob, J.J. and Michaud, G.M. (1976). Production par la naloxone d'effects inverses de ceux, de la morphine chez le chien éveillé. *Archives internationales et Pharmacodynamie et de Thérapie, 222*, 332 – 340.

Jacob, J.J., Tremblay, E.C. and Colombel, M.C. (1974). Facilitation de réactions nociceptives par la naloxone chez la souris et chez le rat. *Psychopharmacologia, 37*, 217 – 223.

Mayer, D.J., Price, D.D. and Rafii, A. (1977). Antagonism of acupuncture analgesia in man by the narcotic antagonist naloxone. *Brain Research,* **121**, 368–372.

Pert, C.B., Pert, A. and Tallman, J.F. (1976). Isolation of a novel endogenous opiate analgesic from human blood. *Proceedings of the National Academy of Sciences, U.S.A.,* **73**, 2226–2230.

# Session 4 Chairman: J. D. P. Graham

# 10. Problems of abuse and dependence on analgesic drugs

T H BEWLEY

Physical dependence is relatively easy to recognise and measure but probably is not an important factor in explaining addiction to, and misuse of, drugs. Psychological dependence may be of greater importance but it is hard to define or to measure except to describe some feeling of desire or craving to use a drug and the behaviour of continuing to seek it. Some drugs which produce neither physical dependence nor psychological dependence can also be misused, for example, L.S.D. This is an interesting example of a drug that few people would have predicted would have been used or misused in the fashion that occurred in the 1960's and 1970's and up to the present. From the pharmacological point of view it does not produce dependence and it is very uncertain in its actions. The effects of taking it can at times be frightening or unpleasant and it is not obvious why the effects that it does produce should prove attractive. The only certain conclusion that can be drawn, is that any psychoactive drug can presumably be liable to misuse by some people.

Human behaviour is complex and often irrational, and this may be more important than other aspects of pharmacology when estimating the misuse liability of a new drug. It is relatively easy to predict that drugs with marked similarity to other dependence producing drugs will likewise produce dependence, but it is very much more difficult to predict this in the case of drugs with unknown properties. It has been suggested that the simplest way to find out if a drug is liable to be misused is to go down and ask the 'boys in the street' if they are currently misusing it, and for their views of its effects, as they can at times be some years ahead of modern psychopharmacology in finding drugs that are suitable for misuse.

People who misuse drugs obtained illicitly are liable to use drugs of all types and many patients who are conveniently classified as heroin or opiate addicts are in practice poly-drug misusers who also take amphetamines and barbiturates. Some of these have much greater problems from the misuse of amphetamines, leading to deterioration in their behaviour, than they do from taking opiates, although the amphetamines do not cause physical dependence.

Oswald (1969) described the effects of taking heroin for sufficiently long to produce dependence, shown by withdrawal symptoms on stopping. He made the point that heroin produced no pleasure for him, more a sense of weariness with at the most 'some hours of disinterest, the world passing by while he felt untouched'. He described the withdrawal symptoms as not bad, merely noticeable with the ever present feeling of weariness that he had before 'just that much worse; a headache, yawning, shiverings and cold feelings, a nose that hurt like a common cold, hands a little shaky and poor in grip'. He stated a month after the experiment that he had begun to reconsider a sociologist's view that it wasn't the withdrawal symptoms or inner pleasures that kept people on heroin but possibly 'social pressure to belong to the group who had taken this famously traditional exit'. Brill (1968) in a paper on misapprehensions about drug addiction pointed out that the pains of withdrawal had been exaggerated as a factor in addiction.

I will briefly review the treatment of opiate dependence in the United Kingdom, which has generally been by prescribing opiates for addicts attending special clinics. I hope to make the point that the clinicians for practical purposes ignore the factor of tolerance, and that physical dependence is only a small part of the problem of addiction and its treatment.

## Goals of treatment
There can be five goals, when treating opiate dependence.

### Abstinence
Total withdrawal from all misuse of drugs and return to normal functioning. This would be an ideal outcome, but in practice will only be achieved in a small number of cases.

### Better functioning
Better functioning despite continued use of drugs. The aim would be to enable a patient to lead a normal life, apart from the use of drugs. This can be measured in terms of social functioning (work record, convictions, housing, family stability) or health complications such as hepatitis, overdoses or abscesses.

### Treatment of complications
If, despite treatment, the patient does badly he is likely to require more medical care for the treatment of overdoses, septic complications and psychoses and social support for his problems.

### Acceptability
Any régime will need to be acceptable to the patient or he will not attend.

### Prevention
By controlling the availability of drugs there should be less likelihood of producing new cases of addiction.

## Prescribing opiates to addicts
When opiates are prescribed for an addict who is dependent on them this can be described as treatment or as crime. Until methadone maintenance clinics were started in the United States, a doctor who prescribed opiates to an addict was liable to be prosecuted. Various reasons for prescribing in this way have been put forward. For many years it was believed that there was a system known as the 'British system'

whereby opiate addicts could have opiates prescribed for them and that this led to the very small number of people dependent on drugs. In fact, there was no system, but as there was very little in the way of misuse of drugs this did not matter (Brill, 1968). Original guide lines for prescribing of opiates to opiate addicts were laid down in the Rolleston Report (Departmental Committee, 1926). Addicts for whom morphine or heroin could be prescribed, included 'persons for whom, after every effort has been made for the cure of addiction, the drug cannot be completely withdrawn, either because:

1.    Complete withdrawal produces serious symptoms which cannot be satisfactorily treated under the ordinary conditions of private (general) practice; or

2.    The patient, while capable of leading a useful and fairly normal life so long as he takes a certain non-progressive quantity, usually small, of the drug of addiction, ceases to be able to do so when the regular allowance is withdrawn'.

Other reasons for using opiates to treat opiate addiction have been put forward; for example, Dole, Nyswander and Kreek (1966) suggested that methadone was an opiate which taken orally and regularly did not produce euphoria, and that if it was taken in sufficient quantities it would 'blockade' the euphoriant effects of heroin,so that a person who was having a regular amount of methadone would have no effects from taking heroin, and no need to seek it. Another model is that of ameliorating the condition by substituting a less harmful for a more harmful type of dependence. This might include substituting methadone for heroin since it is a longer acting opiate. Those who used it would be less likely to have periods when they suffered withdrawal symptoms, since by giving them a regular daily dose there should be no occasion when they would go for a sufficiently long period to have withdrawal symptoms. A different model was used by Dr John Owens (1967),who took the view that opiate dependence was generally associated with a disorder of personality and that both the dependence and the personality disorder were untreatable. He considered that the aim of the treatment should be to prevent new cases developing. This could only be done by dealing with the problem locally and he instituted a system whereby he alone prescribed drugs to all addicts in his area. He worked very closely with the local Drugs Squad and local pharmacists to ensure that all the drugs prescribed went into the patient concerned. He considered that questions of pharmacology were irrelevant and prescribed heroin and cocaine on the grounds that this was what the patients wanted and as long as they didn't give it to anyone else, they would do no harm to anyone except themselves.

Another model, and one which partly underlay the setting up of Treatment Clinics at the end of the 1960's,was that people who had become dependent on drugs were not able to obtain drugs sufficiently easily to cope with life and to prevent withdrawal symptoms since they were unable to get the amount of drugs they needed. It had been suggested (Frankau 1964) that if sufficient drugs were prescribed,they would lose the need to obtain drugs illicitly and would have time to concentrate on returning to a steady and sober way of life. It was hoped that by prescribing sufficient drugs for the patient a good relationship would be established with the therapist,who would later use this with his other therapeutic and psycho-therapeutic arts,to motivate the patient to enter hospital, be weaned off drugs and live happily ever afterwards.

Another suggestion was that all of these were wrong and that the main aim of prescribing drugs was to ensure that a patient would remain in regular contact with medical and social facilities so that treatment could be provided for complications and advice given about life problems. Another model put forward was that prescribing methadone for addicts was not treatment at all, but merely a method whereby society controlled deviants, and a variant of this was that it was part of a method to continue to keep the black community in the United States deferential, defeated and demoralised (Pierce, 1973).

### Maintenance clinics

In the past eight years there have been gradual changes in treatment practice. After the implementation in April, 1968 of the 1967 Dangerous Drugs Act a large number of patients first attended the new clinics where the doctors continued to prescribe for them. Gradually a better assessment was made of individual patients, and generally the amounts prescribed were reduced. Eventually it became easier to assess new patients as to whether they were using drugs or not, and if they were physically dependent. A general system of control was introduced whereby all patients who were having drugs prescribed for them attended at least once a week and were given prescriptions which could be collected daily. The prescriptions were sent to individual chemists made out in such a way that the patient could only get one day's supply of drugs at a time, which has remained the system up to the present. At some of the treatment clinics, routine urine testing for the presence of drugs is done weekly on all patients. In one study, although 95 per cent of patients appeared to use all the drugs prescribed for them, most of the time 40 per cent used other drugs as well (Bewley *et al.*, 1973).

There is some evidence that the system has been of value and helped to contain the problem. The rate at which new cases have appeared has been much less than in the previous decade. This might confirm that the system had some preventive value or it might be that the treatment facilities were set up at a time when an epidemic had passed its peak and that the number of cases would have declined anyway. Both are probably partly true (Hughes *et al*, 1972). The number of addicts known to the Home Office each year, the number in treatment and the number of deaths having increased rapidly in the 1960's, slowed down in the 1970's, suggesting some containment of the problem. For the past seven years the estimated average dose of opiates prescribed in the country as a whole has remained at about 80 mg daily. (Table 10.1).

### Current prescribing policy

Since the St Thomas's Hospital Clinic opened there have been changes at different times in the amounts of drugs prescribed and in the arrangements for dispensing them. Initially, all patients continued with any drugs they had previously received on a prescription, and such drugs as cocaine, methylamphetamine, dexamphetamine, tranquillizers and barbiturates were prescribed. This was slowly changed and the

| Year | Number of Addicts known to Home Office December 31 each year | Average number of outpatients daily DHSS | Average daily prescription of opiates (Grammes) | | | | Estimated average daily dose (mgm) | Death attributed to Drug Dependence on Death Certificate (a) | Addicts known to Home Office |
|---|---|---|---|---|---|---|---|---|---|
| | | | Heroin | Methadone Ampoules | Methadone other | Total | | | |
| 1968 (July – Dec) | – | 1066 | 92 | – | – | – | 86[b] | – | (38) |
| 1969 | 1466 | 1115 | 62 | (c) 29 | (c) 9 | 100 | 90 | 53 | (54) |
| 1970 | 1430 | 1155 | 48 | 31 | 10 | 89 | 77 | 33 | (41) |
| 1971 | 1555 | 1036 | 39 | 32 | 10 | 81 | 78 | 38 | |
| 1972 | 1619 | 1252 | 39 | 39 | 22 | 100 | 80 | 58 | |
| 1973 | 1818 | 1380 | 39 | 52 | 25 | 116 | 84 | 64 | |
| 1974 | 1980 | 1496 | 42 | 59 | 23 | 124 | 83 | 72 | (77) |
| 1975 | 1954 | 1546 | 42 | 57 | 26 | 125 | 81 | – | (69) |
| 1976 (d) | – | 1461 | 36 | 48 | 31 | 115 | 79 | – | |

(a) Hansard  (c) Average for last 5 months of 1969
(b) Heroin only  (d) Average for first 10 months of 1976

Table 10.1. Estimated daily dose of opiates prescribed in the United Kingdom 1968–1976.

prescribing of cocaine, amphetamines and barbiturates was gradually phased out. The amounts of opiates prescribed were reduced and for the majority of patients, methadone replaced heroin. In the past four years there have been no changes in the amounts prescribed for any patient, and none has had an increase in dosage. In the past year all new patients attending the clinic, who have been given a prescription, have had one for oral methadone (d.t.f.). The majority of new patients have a total dosage of 40 mg methadone daily, and those who first attended earlier, an average of 80–90 mg of methadone daily. The amounts prescribed in April, 1977 are shown in Table 10.2.

| Total dosage of opiates prescribed | St Thomas' Hospital Drug Dependence Treatment Clinic | All London Clinics |
|---|---|---|
| Up to 39 mgm | 5 | 184 |
| 40 – 79 mgm | 95 | 405 |
| 80 – 119 mgm | 39 | 168 |
| 120 – 199 mgm | 19 | 113 |
| 200 – 499 mgm | 3 | 58 |
| 500 + | 1 | 12 |
| | Total 162 | Total 940 |

Table 10.2. Average daily prescription of opiates (heroin and/or methadone) April 1977.

There were 192 patients currently attending the clinic. (162 patients now having a prescription for an opiate, 11 attended for some other treatment, 12 were temporarily in prison and seven in hospital). 162 patients were having methadone prescribed, and five were having heroin prescribed as well, but heroin is gradually being replaced by methadone as none of those on heroin were benefiting from this. There were only 12 patients whose prescriptions for total opiates were more than 120 mg. a day, and this is being reduced to a maximum of 120 mg, since there is no evidence that being stabilised at any one level is better than any other level. The amounts prescribed to patients having more than 120 mg daily is shown in Table 10.3.

| | Sex | Age | Heroin 10 mgm tabs. I.V. or I.M. | Methadone 10 mgm ampoules I.V. or I.M. | Methadone 5 mgm tabs. orally | Methadone mixture D.T.F. oral:liquid | Total dose of opiates |
|---|---|---|---|---|---|---|---|
| A | Female | | 660 | – | – | – | 660 |
| B | Male | | 60 | 200 | – | – | 260 |
| C | Male | | – | 100 | 100 | – | 200 |
| D | Male | | 180 | 20 | – | – | 200 |
| E | Male | | – | – | 195 | – | 195 |
| F | Male | | – | 170 | – | – | 170 |
| G | Male | | – | 60 | – | 90 | 150 |
| H | Female | | 80 | 60 | | | 140 |
| I.J.K. | Males | | – | 140 | – | – | 140 |
| L | Male | | 100 | 20 | – | – | 120 |

Table 10.3. Amount of opiate prescribed at St Thomas' Hospital having more than 120 mg daily.

All new patients are now given a prescription for oral methadone and the next change will be to prescribe oral methadone to patients who have been off drugs, having been away from the clinic for some time.

## Follow-up study

Wiepert (1977) examined the current status of all opiate addicts treated at two clinics in London. Prescriptions were given to 575 patients, 120 female and 455 male, for periods ranging up to 94 months. In 1975, 52 per cent were still in treatment, 258 at the clinics and 42 elsewhere, 28 per cent were not in treatment, 11 per cent had died, 6 per cent were in custody and 3 per cent had left the country. Consistency of treatment for many patients was striking, with 61 per cent never interrupting treatment. In-patient hospitalisation for drug abuse occurred for 28 per cent. 46 per cent of patients in treatment at clinics at the end of the study were working regularly, an increase from 23 per cent at entry. Not all patients were able to lead relatively stable lives since those treated in hospital for abuse had an average of 8.7 hospitalisations. 11 per cent of patients died, with 51 deaths directly or secondarily attributable to the misuse of drugs. The rate of patients leaving and remaining out of treatment throughout the time period studied remained constant. 7 per cent left in the same year as entry and 8 per cent left after five years, with the rate remaining between 7 and 8 per cent for the years in between. The death rate was found to be between 2 and 3 per cent for all years of treatment except for the first year (Table 10.4.). The drug careers of patients showed that the mean age of first drug use was 17.1 years with treatment beginning at a mean age of 23.6 years. The time between mean age of first use and entry into treatment was 6.5 years for all patients. Wiepert thought that the facts in this study suggested that addiction was a chronic condition with a regular non-episodic

Death rate 1968 – 1975

| Year | Entering each year | In treatment | Current status in October, 1975 | | | | Follow up | |
| | | | Not in treatment | Dead | In Custody | Out of Country | Length in years | Cumulative numbers followed up |
| --- | --- | --- | --- | --- | --- | --- | --- | --- |
| 1968 | 185 | 73 | 59 | 30 | 12 | 11 | 7/8 | 185 |
| 1969 | 87 | 107 | 94 | 40 | 17 | 14 | 6/7 | 272 |
| 1970 | 60 | 132 | 116 | 50 | 19 | 15 | 5/6 | 332 |
| 1971 | 75 | 186 | 132 | 53 | 19 | 17 | 4/5 | 407 |
| 1972 | 71 | 229 | 149 | 60 | 23 | 17 | 3/4 | 478 |
| 1973 | 48 | 263 | 156 | 63 | 26 | 18 | 2/3 | 526 |
| 1974 | 27 | 281 | 160 | 64 | 30 | 18 | 1/2 | 553 |
| 1975 | 22 | 300 | 161 | 64 | 32 | 18 | less than 1 | 575 |

Table 10.4. Details of patients entering, leaving and remaining on treatment, 1968–1975, including number of deaths.

pattern of treatment for many patients, with significant proportions working regularly and with control of their use of injectable opiates. Others were unable to control their use with frequent hospitalisation, and this group had a much higher rate of death than usual for their age group, principally attributable to drug abuse.

## A comparison of injectable heroin and oral methadone

Dr Martin Mitcheson (1977) carried out a clinical trial comparing the prescribing of oral methadone with the prescribing of injectable heroin. The clinical trial was by random allocation. 96 out of 260 opiate users presenting for treatment to University College Hospital between February, 1972 and February, 1974 were selected for a comparison of maintenance with either injectable heroin or oral methadone. All the trial patients had requested heroin and had been accepted by staff as confirmed heroin addicts. The cases were allocated at random to the two treatments with an initial bias to oral methadone. 44 received heroin; 52 were offered only oral methadone. During the year four cases were crossed over from oral methadone to injectable drugs and omitted from subsequent follow-up.

The major outcome of the trial was that in the twelfth month, 32 per cent of those offered methadone and 10 per cent of those offered heroin were consuming on average less than 5 mg of opiates daily. At this time 57 per cent of those offered methadone and 90 per cent of those offered heroin were injecting regularly. During the final three months, 20 per cent of those offered oral methadone abstained from injecting voluntarily for at least 31 days compared to 5 per cent of those having heroin prescribed, and a further 28 per cent of those offered oral methadone abstained for from between three and 30 days compared to 12 per cent of those having heroin prescribed. During the year 50 per cent of those having heroin prescribed and 70 per cent of those having oral methadone prescribed were convicted of a crime. There was no difference between the two groups in terms of employment (62 per cent unemployed) or health. The oral methadone group tended to polarise towards high or low categories in terms of involvement with the drug sub-culture, consumption of non-prescribed (illicit) opiates and criminal activity, whereas the heroin group continued with intermediate levels of involvement with the drug sub-culture, illegal drug use and crime. Not prescribing heroin led to a significantly lower attendance rate at the clinic by the end of the year. At 12 months 76 per cent of those having heroin prescribed and 29 per cent of those having oral methadone prescribed were attending the clinic regularly. 74 per cent of those on heroin and 29 per cent of those on oral methadone were receiving a prescription at 12 month follow-up. Over all, prescribing heroin appeared to maintain the *status quo* with the majority of heroin maintained patients continuing to inject heroin regularly. Prescribing heroin was not associated with any improvement in social functioning or reduction in consumption of illegal drugs, though it might reduce the degree of involvement in criminal activity especially in terms of arrest and conviction rates. Prescribing oral methadone led to a higher abstinence rate. The most striking finding from this study was that there were not very marked differences in outcome between the two groups. The study did not attempt to answer the question whether methadone was a better or worse drug for maintenance therapy of opiate addiction than heroin nor whether oral drugs were better than drugs prescribed for injection. In order to do this it would have been necessary to have a third group who had methadone prescribed to be taken by injection. However, since there was so little difference between oral methadone and injectable heroin it would not seem likely that any great difference would be discovered if either of these were to be compared with methadone prescribed to be taken by injection.

### Development of tolerance and relief of pain

Twycross (1975) reviewed the use of narcotic analgesics in terminal illness in a group of 500 patients admitted to St Christopher's Hospice. To achieve and maintain pain relief, many of the patients received diamorphine (heroin) regularly every four hours. Almost all the patients received a phenothiazine concurrently and other drugs when indicated. He concluded that:

1.  Although most patients received parenteral diamorphine during their last 12 to 24 hours, the majority could be maintained on oral medication until this time.
2.  There was no single optimal dose of diamorphine.
3.  Psychological dependence did not occur.
4.  Physical dependence might develop but did not prevent the downward adjustment of diamorphine when considered clinically feasible.
5.  Tolerance was not a practical problem.
6.  The prescription of diamorphine did not by itself lead to impairment of mental faculties.

He thought it was possible but by no means certain that many of the 205 patients who received diamorphine for more than one week became physically dependent on it. Eddy and his associates (1959) had previously reviewed cancer patients maintained on subcutaneous morphine, oxymorphine and anileridine and had tested for physical dependence by injecting nalorphine hydrochloride 1 mg subcutaneously at fortnightly intervals. They had shown that over half the patients developed physical dependence by the end of the second week of treatment and that it was unusual for a patient not to be physically dependent by the end of the fourth week. All the patients were receiving morphine by injection. Twycross (1975) concluded that whether or not physical dependence developed it did not prevent the gradual downward adjustment of dose nor the complete curtailment of treatment when this became clinically feasible. The data in his review, especially those relating to patients who survived for 24 weeks or more after commencing treatment with diamorphine, supported the hypothesis that increases in dose were caused more by increased pain than by tolerance. It would be possible to induce marked tolerance by needlessly increasing a dose, but he found no support for the statement that due to tolerance, morphine would cease to be effective after three months of continuous use. In practice, when diamorphine was used at St Christopher's Hospice regularly, prophylactically and as part of a programme of total care, tolerance, if it occurred, was not a practical problem.

## Conclusions

It is possible to prescribe opiates for very long periods in the treatment of pain, and also to sustain addiction without difficulty, and without having to continually escalate the dosage because of the development of tolerance. It is possible to increase the amounts prescribed for addicts in such a way that they develop tolerance to very large doses, but it is not desirable to do this. Prescribing opiates to addicts who are dependent on them is a method of treatment which appears to lead to some improvement (measured by general stability and social functioning) if it is done in a carefully controlled way. Uncontrolled prescribing of opiates to addicts appeared to lead to a marked increase in their numbers in this country 10 years ago. There is no evidence to suggest that prescribing either heroin or methadone (whether by injection or orally) makes much difference to the outcome. In the circumstances clinicians now are more likely to prescribe oral methadone for new patients, who come for maintenance treatment for their addiction. The reason for this is to make addiction boring, dull, steady, safe and square, rather than seeing it in terms of sin, vice, crime, degradation and risk.

### References

Bewley, T.H., James, I.P., Le Fevre, C., Maddocks, P. & Mahon, T. (1973). Maintenance treatment of narcotic addicts. *The International Journal of the Addictions.* 7, No.4, 597–612.
Brill, H. (1968). Misapprehensions about drug addiction; some origins and repercussions. *Comprehensive Psychiatry,* (1968) 4, 150–159.
Dole, V.P., Nyswander, M.E. & Kreek, M.J. (1966). Narcotic Blockade. *Archives of Internal Medicine,* 118, 304–309.
Eddy, N.B., Lee, L.E., Harris, C.A. (1959). The rate of development of physical dependence and tolerance to analgesic drugs in patients with chronic pain. *Bulletin on Narcotics,* 11, 3–17.

Frankau, I.M. (1964). Treatment in England of Canadian patients addicted to narcotic drugs. *Canadian Medical Association Journal,* **90**, 421 – 424.

Hughes, P.H., Barker, N.W., Crawford, G.A., Jaffe, J.H. (1972). The natural history of a heroin epidemic. *American Journal of Public Health,* 995–1001.

Ministry of Health. Departmental Committee (Rolleston Committee) (1926). *Report of the Departmental Committee on Morphine and Heroin Addiction,* London, H.M.S.O.

Mitcheson, M., (1977). A controlled trial of heroin and methadone in the treatment of opiate dependence. Personal Communication. Submitted for publication *Archives General Psychiatry.*

Owens, J. (1967). Centres for treatment of drug addiction : integrated approach. *British Medical Journal.* **2**, 501–455.

Oswald, I. (1969). Personal view. *British Medical Journal,* **1**, 438.

Pierce, C.M. (1973). Race, deprivation and drug abuse in the U.S.A. in: *Anglo American Conference on Drug Abuse:* London: Royal Society of Medicine, pp. 69–76.

Twycross, R.G. (1975). The use of narcotic analgesics in terminal illness. *Journal of Medical Ethics,* (1975) **1**, 10–17.

Wiepert, G.D. (1977). A follow-up of 575 British opiate addicts in treatment for eight years. Personal communication; awaiting submission for publication.

# 11. The assessment of abuse potential drugs of the opiate type

J. D. P. GRAHAM AND J. W. LEWIS

We are all painfully aware of the personal and social harm which can be visited upon him who seeks relief by means of addictive drugs. One of us (JDPG) has just returned from an inspection of the treatment facilities offered by the Government and the Voluntary Agencies of Hong Kong to the 50—100,000 persons there who are dependent upon heroin. Courageous as is the effort made, it only deals with a small minority of the victims. Dr Bewley has reviewed the situation as he finds it today in the United Kingdom; we have all heard of the epidemic state of heroin abuse in North America. It goes without saying that when a new drug of the class of 'strong analgesic' is presented for clinical use, we examine it with care as to its addiction potential. Before we can make a rational judgement it is necessary to comprehend the methodology applied to answering the question, and to have an informed opinion on the validity of the tests applied and the relative emphasis to be placed on these tests. Our record in the past is not a fit subject for complacency, and it is probably wise to speak in relative terms of any new narcotic, using morphine as our yardstick.

Psychoactive drugs which obtund the sensation of pain are liable to have abuse potential. This can be tested for in animal models and in man. While the former is essential in order to gain preliminary information it is in man that the crucial tests must be made and it is from ongoing clinical experience that the final answer comes, usually after a number of years of widespread legitimate use. The subject has been reviewed in detail recently (Committee on Problems of Drug Dependence, 1973). Drugs which have abuse potential usually display one or more of the following characteristics:-

1.  Tolerance
2.  Physical dependence
3.  Drug seeking behaviour and reinforcement
    (Psychological dependence)
4.  Negative reinforcement on withdrawal


## Tolerance

Tolerance is easy to demonstrate in laboratory animals. The crude but precise endpoint of lethality may be used. If the LD50 of a drug is greatly increased on repetitive dosing, tolerance has been induced. More subtle but not necessarily more rewarding data may be obtained from one of a host of behavioural models.

## Physical dependence

If the drug has a capacity to induce physical dependence there will be a recognisable and reproducible syndrome on withdrawal of the drug following chronic administration and this may be precipitated or enhanced by challenge with naloxone, a specific narcotic antagonist. Moreover, a drug that will suppress the withdrawal syndrome in abstinent morphine-dependent subjects can be classified as supporting morphine-like physical dependence.

Mice may be made dependent on morphine or a test drug by repeated administration of the drug or, more conveniently, by implantation of a pellet which slowly releases the drug (Hui and Roberts, 1975). The detection of the level of dependence induced is made by challenge with the antagonists nalorphine or naloxone. In mice treated with drugs of high dependence liability nalorphine and naloxone produce an abstinence syndrome, the most characteristic sign of which is compulsive jumping (Maggiolo and Huidobro, 1961).Naloxone challenge to animals treated with drugs of intermediate dependence liability produces jumping of limited extent.

In the best developed technique for producing physical dependence in rats, morphine or the test drug is infused via an intraperitoneal cannula over a period of up to six days (Teiger, 1974). When the infusion of morphine is stopped a characteristic abstinence syndrome develops over the first twenty-four hours which includes weight loss (20 per cent), 'wet dog shakes', diarrhoea, squealing, hyperirritability, aggressiveness, rubbing and chewing (Teiger, 1974). The weight loss and hyperirritability appear to be the most reproducible effects. The level of the abstinence syndrome from a test drug can be compared with that from morphine, and in addition, the ability of the test drug to precipitate abstinence or to substitute for morphine can be judged by replacing morphine by the test drug in the infusion solution (Teiger, 1976).

The chronic 'spinal' dog, is a model for dependence studies which has proved to be particularly sensitive and to give good correlation with results in man, as developed by Martin (Martin et al., 1974). In dogs which have been subjected to cord transection of level T10–T11, two significant spinal reflexes can be recorded, viz (a) limb flexion in response to pressure, (b) skin twitch in response to thermal stimulus. The morphine abstinence syndrome in this model is characterised by a number of non-measurable signs of which retching and emesis are the most significant. In addition there are graded signs such as lacrimation, salivation and tremor, and measurable signs — pupil dilation, increase of pulse rate and respiratory rate, decrease of threshold for the skin twitch and enhancement of the amplitude of the stimulated flexor reflex.

The abuse potential of narcotic analgesics and antagonist-analgesics can be assessed in monkeys in terms of morphine-substitution, primary physical dependence and drug-seeking reinforcing effects; Yanagita has reviewed all these aspects (Yanagita, 1973). The morphine abstinence syndrome in rhesus monkeys is classified into graded levels as follows (Committee on Problems of Drug Dependence, 1973):

*Mild:* Apprehension, continual yawning, rhinorrhoea, lacrimation, hiccup, shivering, perspiration on face, chattering, quarrelling and fighting.

*Intermediate:* Tremor, anorexia, pilomotor activity, muscle twitching and rigidity and holding the abdomen (cramps).

*Severe:* Extreme restlessness, assumption of peculiar attitudes, vomiting, severe diarrhoea, erection and continued masturbation, inflammation of the eyelids and conjunctivae (insomnia), continual calling and crying, lying on side with eyes closed and marked spasticity.

*Very severe:* Docility in the normally excitable animal, dyspnoea, pallor, strabismus, dehydration, weight loss, prostration, circulatory collapse and, occasionally, death.

Morphine dependence is maintained by subcutaneous administration of 3 mg/kg of morphine sulphate every six hours. In substitution tests, morphine is withheld until the development of an abstinence syndrome of intermediate intensity (about 14 hours): administration of a test morphine-like drug at this time will partially or completely suppress the abstinence syndrome.

In primary physical dependence studies in rhesus monkeys, the highest tolerable dose of the test drug is administered for at least 31 days at intervals (two–six hours) related to the drug's duration of action. The development of physical dependence is monitored at the twenty-eighth day by the administration of nalorphine and/or naloxone. The severity of any abstinence syndrome produced by this challenge indicates the level of physical dependence. After termination of drug treatment the monkeys are observed for withdrawal reactions.

In mice, rats, dogs and rhesus monkeys, morphine antagonist properties in a test drug can be identified by its ability to precipitate an abstinence syndrome in morphine-dependent animals. In each of these tests it is possible to estimate the potency of the test drug relative to a standard, usually nalorphine or naloxone.

The procedure for assessment of dependence liability in man at the Addiction Research Centre, Lexington, Kentucky, used volunteer male prisoners who were former opiate addicts; sociological and political pressures have very recently stopped the use of this class of subject. In single-dose, double-blind studies, changes in physiological parameters and subjective assessment by the subjects were used to compare test drugs with morphine and, if appropriate, nalorphine. This comparison was used to make an assessment of the reinforcing properties of the test drug (Committee on Problems of Drug Dependence, 1973).

Substitution for morphine was assessed in subjects dependent on stabilisation doses of either 60 mg or 240 mg morphine sulphate per day. The morphine abstinence syndrome was characterised and quantified on the Himmelsbach scale (Table 11.1, Kolb and Himmelsbach, 1938). Suppression of abstinence by a test drug was measured by reduction of the Himmelsbach score. Whereas drugs of high dependence liability suppressed abstinence in both '240 mg' and '60 mg' groups, certain partial agonists with limited morphine-like activity showed morphine antagonist activity in the '240 mg' group by precipitating abstinence in the non-withdrawn subjects, whilst substituting for morphine in withdrawn '60 mg' subjects (Jasinski, Martin and Hoeldtke, 1971).

Direct dependence studies at the Addiction Research Centre used a schedule similar to that used in the rhesus monkey model. The effects of nalorphine or naloxone challenge and abrupt withdrawal were evaluated on the Himmelsbach scale (Committee on Problems of Drug Dependence, 1973).

In the monkey, dog and man, antagonist analgesics of the nalorphine-cyclazocine type produce primary physical dependence which is manifest as abstinence syndrome qualitatively different from the morphine-abstinence syndromes in these models. For example, Martin and his collaborators (Martin and Gorodetsky, 1965) showed that

Table 11.1. Himmelsbach abstinence scoring system (The score for any 24-hour day is the sum of these points.

A.  Signs accurately measurable

Fever: one point for each 0.1°C (rectal) rise.
Hyperpnea: one point for each respiration/minute increase.
Systolic blood pressure: one point for each 2 mm Hg rise (up to 30 mm).
Weight: one point for each pound loss.

B.  Signs not accurately measurable

| | |
|---|---|
| Yawning<br>Lacrimation<br>Rhinorrhea<br>Perspiration | one point only for any of these signs<br>observed on any one day |
| Anorexia<br>Goose flesh<br>Dilated pupils<br>Tremor | three points only for any of these signs<br>observed on any one day |
| Restlessness | five points only in one day |
| Emesis | five points for each emesis observed |

in man the proportion of points from the Himmelsbach abstinence score differs for morphine and nalorphine. The most important sources of points in the morphine syndrome were hyperpnoea and increase of blood pressure whereas for nalorphine most points came from increase in body temperature and weight loss. Other antagonist analgesics such as pentazocine show syndromes which have characteristics of both morphine and nalorphine abstinence.

## Reinforcing properties

Several approaches to the assessment of reinforcement of drug-seeking behaviour (psychological dependence) in monkeys using self-administration techniques have been used (Yanagita, 1973),e.g. (*a*) making the drug available to the naive animal for spontaneous initiation and continuation of self administration (*b*) assessment of the response to the drug after sustained self-administration of a known reinforcing drug. In these tests all compounds with an appreciable level of morphine-like activity demonstrate drug-seeking behaviour. Drugs of the antagonist-analgesic class with predominant agonist effects,e.g. pentazocine and propiram,also display positive reinforcing properties,whereas predominantly antagonist drugs such as nalorphine and cyclazocine are negative reinforcers since rates of self administration for these drugs are below the saline level (Hoffmeister and Wuttke, 1974).

## Dependence profiles of some drugs of relatively low abuse potential

The development of sensitive tests for abuse potential has been encouraged by the evolution of new strong analgesic agents having lower dependence producing potential than morphine. Typical of this class are d-propoxyphene, pentazocine, propiram, nalorphine, butorphanol and buprenorphine, the structures of which are shown in Figure 11.1. Most of these compounds have been studied in rhesus monkeys at the University of Michigan, and in the chronic 'spinal' dog (Martin *et al.,* 1974) and man (Committee on Problems of Drug Dependence, 1973) at the Addiction Research Centre, Lexington, so that comparison of their potential for producing dependence can be made from data generated in these studies. The results of the animal studies are shown in Tables 11.2 and 11.3 and the human studies in Table 11.4.

Table 11.2. Results of dependence studies in the Morphine-dependent chronic spinal dog.

| Compound | Withdrawn | Non-withdrawn | Ref. |
|---|---|---|---|
| Propoxyphene | Suppn. | NT | 13 |
| Pentazocine | No suppn. | Pptn. | 16 |
| Propiram | Suppn. | Pptn. | 16 |
| Nalbuphine | NT | NT | |
| Butorphanol | NT | NT | |
| Buprenorphine | Partial suppn. | Pptn. | 13 |

Suppn = suppression of abstinence.
Pptn = precipitation of abstinence.

Table 11.3. Results of dependence studies in the Rhesus Monkey.

| Compound | M—dependent | Ref. | Direct dependence | | | |
|---|---|---|---|---|---|---|
| | | | Nalorphine | Naloxone | Withdrawal | Ref. |
| Propoxyphene | Suppn. | 7 | NT | NT | ++ | 7 |
| Pentazocine | Pptn. | 15 | ± | + | + | 17 |
| Propiram | Pptn. | 18 | NT | NT | ++ | 7 |
| Nalbuphine | Pptn. | 20 | 0 | ++ | ++ | 21 |
| Butorphanol | No suppn. | 28 | NT | NT | NT | |
| Buprenorphine | Pptn. | 27 | 0 | 0 | 0 | 26 |

M = Morphine; Suppn = suppression of abstinence in withdrawn animals,
Pptn = precipitation of abstinence in non-withdrawn animals.
Results of direct dependence tests refer to intensity of abstinence precipitated by antagonists and on abrupt withdrawal.

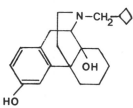

**Propoxyphene**

**Propiram**

**Pentazocine**

**Nalbuphine**

**Butorphanol**

**Buprenorphine**

Fig. 11.1.

Table 11.4. Results of dependence studies in man at the Addiction Research Centre, Lexington, Ky. Morphine-like euphoria assessed from MBG score. Nalorphine-like effects from PCAG and LSD scores. Suppression of M–abstinence assessed in withdrawn subject, precipitation in non-withdrawn subjects. Precipitation of abstinence in direct dependence studies scored as +. NT = not tested.

| Compound | Subjective effects | | Effects in M-dependent subjects | | Direct dependence | | |
|---|---|---|---|---|---|---|---|
| | Maximal M-like euphoria | Nalorphine-like effects | 60 mg | 240 mg | Nalorphine challenge | Naloxone challenge | Ref. |
| Propoxyphene | +++ | 0 | NT | Suppn. | + | NT | 12 |
| Pentazocine | + | +++ | No suppn. | Pptn. | 0 | + | 14 |
| Propiram | +++ | + | Suppn. | Pptn. | + | NT | 9 |
| Nalbuphine | + | + | Pptn. | Pptn. | 0 | + | 19 |
| Butorphanol | + | ++ | Mild Pptn. | NT | + | + | 22, 23 |
| Buprenorphine | ++ | 0 | NT | NT | NT | 0 | 23 |

Propoxyphene displayed the profile of a morphine-like agonist without any antagonist properties. It showed the full range of morphine subjective effects in man (Fraser and Isbell, 1960) and suppressed abstinence in withdrawn morphine-dependent dogs (Martin *et al.*, 1976), monkeys (Yanagita, 1973) and man (Fraser and Isbell, 1960). In the latter, the level of physical dependence attained by chronic administration of d-propoxyphene was limited by the inability to raise the daily dosage above a level equivalent to 60 mg morphine due to the low toxicity threshold.

Of the substances under review, pentazocine showed the highest level of nalorphine-like effects in its profile. At lower doses in man (Jasinski, Martin and Hoeldtke, 1970), pentazocine was predominantly morphine-like; the maximum level of morphine-like euphoria achieved with single doses of pentazocine corresponded to a dose of 10 mg morphine. At higher doses, dysphoric effects normally associated with nalorphine, but not morphine, became evident. Pentazocine is a weak narcotic antagonist which in monkey (Villarreal and Karbowski, 1974), dog (Gilbert and Martin, 1976) and man (Jasinki, Martin and Hoeldtke, 1970) precipitated abstinence in non-withdrawn morphine-dependent subjects, and did not suppress abstinence in withdrawn morphine-dependent subjects. In direct dependence studies with pentazocine in rhesus monkeys (Swain and Seevers, 1976), nalorphine precipitated a mild abstinence syndrome and naloxone precipitated a moderate syndrome, which was also produced on abrupt withdrawal. The signs of abstinence were qualitatively different from those following withdrawal of morphine and resembled the signs of cyclazocine or nalorphine abstinence. In man the direct dependence study (Jasinski, Martin and Hoeldtke, 1970) of pentazocine gave results generally similar to those obtained in the rhesus monkey, but nalorphine failed to precipitate an abstinence syndrome. The syndrome following abrupt withdrawal included drug-seeking behaviour.

Propiram showed predominantly morphine-like characteristics but there was evidence for a ceiling to these effects in man at the level of a dose of 30 mg of morphine (Jasinski, Martin and Hoeldtke, 1971). Propiram was shown to be a morphine antagonist by precipitation of abstinence in morphine-dependent monkeys (Villareal and Seevers, 1967), chronic 'spinal' dogs (Gilbert and Martin, 1976) and in addicted humans stabilised at 240 mg morphine per day (Jasinski, Martin and Hoeldtke, 1971). At a lower level of morphine dependence (60 mg per day) in man, propiram substituted for morphine in withdrawn subjects, as it did in the withdrawn dependent chronic 'spinal' dog (Gilbert and Martin, 1976). In substituting for morphine in these tests and in showing only a very low level of nalorphine-like subjective effects, propiram differed from pentazocine. In a direct dependence study of propiram in man (Jasinski, Martin and Hoeldtke, 1971), nalorphine precipitated a mild abstinence syndrome which was also produced following abrupt withdrawal of the drug; more drug was requested to relieve this discomfort.

Nalbuphine showed similarity to pentazocine in failing, under all tested circumstances, to suppress morphine abstinence and in showing consistent morphine antagonist properties (Jasinski and Mansky, 1972; Villarreal and Seevers, 1968). The maximum level of morphine-like euphoria achievable by nalbuphine in man was, like pentazocine, only at the level corresponding to 10 mg of morphine, but the level of nalorphine-like effects was a good deal lower than that of pentazocine (Jasinski and Mansky, 1972). In the direct dependence study of nalbuphine in man naloxone, but not nalorphine, produced a definite abstinence syndrome. Following abrupt withdrawal there was produced a moderate abstinence syndrome qualitatively similar to, but of greater intensity than that following withdrawal of pentazocine (Jasinski and Mansky, 1972). In the direct dependence study of nalbuphine in the rhesus monkey, naloxone but not nalorphine precipitated abstinence and, surprisingly, the abstinence syndrome following abrupt withdrawal was morphine-like and classified as of 'high intensity' (Villarreal and Seevers, 1968).

The profile of butorphanol in the dependence models was similar to those of pentazocine and nalbuphine. Its nalorphine-like subjective effects in man were somewhat less pronounced than those of pentazocine but greater than those of nalbuphine (Jasinski et al, 1973). It did not suppress morphine abstinence in any of the models but produced primary physical dependence in man which was associated with an abstinence syndrome more nalorphine-like than morphine-like (Jasinski et al, 1976). Surprisingly abstinence was precipitated by nalorphine as well as by naloxone.

The profile of buprenorphine in the dependence models in some ways resembled that of propiram but there were very important differences. In the morphine-dependent chronic 'spinal' dog (Martin et al, 1976) buprenorphine precipitated abstinence in non-withdrawn animals and partially suppressed abstinence in withdrawn animals. The slope of the dose-response curve for suppression was less than that of morphine and propiram, so that it was concluded that buprenorphine had a lower maximal level of morphine-like agonist activity than either of these agents. Buprenorphine showed extremely long lasting morphine-like subjective effects in man with a ceiling at the 20-30 mg morphine level (Jasinski et al, 1976). There was no evidence of psychotomimetic effects which are characteristic of higher doses of pentazocine and, to a less extent, nalbuphine. Though substitution and precipitation studies in morphine-dependent subjects were not undertaken at Lexington there is evidence from other sources of the narcotic antagonist activity of buprenorphine in man. Abstinence was precipitated by treatment of cancer patients tolerant to narcotics with buprenorphine (Houde *et al*, 1976) and reversal of fentanyl used in anaesthesia by buprenorphine has also been reported (De Castro and Parmentier, 1976).

The main differences between buprenorphine and the other agents were shown in direct dependence studies. In the rhesus monkey (Swain and Seevers, 1975) no abstinence signs were seen on nalorphine or naloxone challenge nor following abrupt withdrawal. The low level of primary dependence produced in the chronic 'spinal' dog (Martin *et al*, 1976) cannot be compared with the other agents since none of the latter have been evaluated in this model. In the direct dependence study of buprenorphine in man (Jasinski *et al.*, 1976), naloxone failed to induce an abstinence syndrome. Figure 11.2 shows the dose-response curve for naloxone precipitation in subjects who received a low stabilisation dose (30 mg/day) of morphine and the full stabilisation

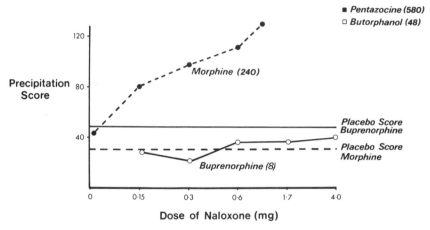

Fig. 11.2. Abstinence scores following the administration of placebo and naloxone to subjects dependent on morphine, 30 mg daily (closed circles), buprenorphine, 8 mg daily (open circles), butorphanol, 48 mg daily, (open square), and pentazocine, 580 mg daily, (closed squares).

dose of buprenorphine (8 mg/day), together with single points for precipitation in subjects stabilised on butorphanol and pentazocine. On abrupt withdrawal the buprenorphine abstinence syndrome was of an extremely mild nature which, during the first two weeks, did not give rise to requests for more drug, and was classified as below the level of clinical significance for morphine withdrawal. Comparison of the abstinence scores on withdrawal of a number of analgesic agents, including all but propoxyphene of the compounds under review, is made in Table 11.5. The score for buprenorphine for the first 10 days following withdrawal of the drug was lower than that for any other clinically effective analgesic agent studied at Lexington.

A surprising feature of the dependence profile of buprenorphine in man (Jasinski *et al*, 1976) was that 14 days after withdrawal of the drug the abstinence syndrome suddenly increased from extremely mild to a level (classified as mild) similar to the maximum level shown by propiram, and subjects demanded morphine to relieve their distress. It would appear that buprenorphine was available for receptor occupation

Table 11.5. Comparison of peak and total area Himmelsbach scores for the first 10 days of withdrawal of strong analgesic agents.

| Drug | Daily Dose | Number of subjects | Potency | Morphine equivalence | Total abstinence scores | Peak score |
|------|-----------|--------------------|---------|----------------------|-------------------------|------------|
| Morphine | 240 mg | 8 | 1 | 240 mg | $198.1 \pm 16.3$ | $36.8 \pm 2.7$ |
| Nalbuphine | 203 mg | 5 | 5/4 | 243 mg | $136.0 \pm 6.4$ | $24.4 \pm 1.5$ |
| Pentazocine | 580 mg | 6 | 1/4 | 145 mg | $106.0 \pm 9.3$ | $15.8 \pm 1.8$ |
| Butorphanol | 48 mg | 6 | 5 | 240 mg | $164.1 \pm 15.2$ | $26.3 \pm 3.7$ |
| Propiram | 1786 mg | 3 | 1/8 | 222 mg | $129.5 \pm 32.0$ | $21.3 \pm 3.4$ |
| Buprenorphine | 8 mg | 5 | 30 | 240 mg | $61.3 \pm 4.2$ | $11.0 \pm 2.6$ |

for this long period after withdrawal of the drug; confirmation of this was obtained from measurements of pupillary diameter (Jasinski et al., 1976).

In summary, propoxyphene is a typical morphine-like agent whose abuse is limited by toxic side effects whereas pentazocine, nalbuphine, butorphanol, propiram and buprenorphine are all antagonist-analgesics with limited morphine-like effects. Pentazocine, nalbuphine and butorphanol will not substitute for morphine in morphine-dependent subjects whereas there are circumstances in which propiram and buprenorphine will. On this basis propiram and buprenorphine have been classified as partial agonists at the morphine ($\mu$) receptor, whereas pentazocine, nalbuphine and butorphanol, like nalorphine, are believed to exert their agonist actions at the ketocyclazocine (kappa) receptor (Martin et al., 1976).

It has been concluded that the abuse potential of partial agonists is greater than that of (kappa) partial agonists. This conclusion may not be true in the case of buprenorphine since, following repeated dosing in man, the level of acute abstinence produced by naloxone precipitation or abrupt withdrawal is much lower than that produced following repeated dosing of pentazocine, nalbuphine or butorphanol.

### References

Committee on Problems of Drug Dependence, (1973) Testing for dependence liability in animals and man (Revised 1972), *Bulletin of Narcotics*, **25**, 25–39.

De Castro, J. and Parmentier, P. (1976) Utilisation of buprenorphine in analgesic anaesthesia, Presented at VI World Congress of Anaesthesiology, Mexico City, Section 5, Sub-section 5.

Fraser, H.F., and Isbell, H. (1960) Pharmacology and addiction liability of dl and d-propoxyphene, *Bulletin of Narcotics*, **12**, 15–23.

Gilbert, P.E. and Martin, W.R. (1976) The effects of morphine and nalorphine-like drugs in the non-dependent, morphine-dependent and cyclazocine-dependent chronic 'spinal' dog. *Journal of Pharmacology and experimental Therapeutics*, **198**, 66–82.

Hoffmeister, F., and Wuttke, W. (1974) Self administration: Positive and negative reinforcing properties of morphine antagonists in rhesus monkeys. *Narcotic Antagonists, Advances in Biochemical Psychopharmacology*, **8**, 361–369. Raven Press, New York.

Houde, R.W., Wallenstein, S.L., Rogers, A., and Kaiko, R.F., (1976): Personal communication as reported to the Committee on Problems of Drug Dependence, National Research Council.

Hui, K.S. and Roberts, M.B. (1975): An improved implantation pellet for the rapid induction of morphine dependence in mice, *Journal of Pharmacy and Pharmacology*, **27**, 569–573.

Jasinski, D.R., Martin, W.R., and Hoeldtke, R.D. (1970): Effects of short and long-term administration of pentazocine in man. *Clinical Pharmacology and Therapeutics*. **11**, 385–403.

94

Jasinski, D.R., Martin, W.R., and Hoeldtke, R. (1971): Studies of the dependence-producing potential of GPA-1657, profadol and propiram in man. *Clinical Pharmacology and Therapeutics.* **12**, 613–649.

Jasinski, D.R. and Mansky, P.A. (1972): Evaluation of nalbuphine for abuse potential. *Clinical Pharmacology and Therapeutics.* **13**, 78–90.

Jasinski, D.R., Griffith, J.D. Prevnick, J.S., and Clark, S.C. (1975): Personal communication as reported to the Committee on Problems of Drug Dependence, National Research Council.

Jasinski, D.R., Prevnick, J.S., Griffith, J.D., Gorodetzky, C.W. and Cone, E.J. (1976): Personal communication as reported to the Committee on Problems of Drug Dependence, National Research Council.

Kolb, L. and Himmelsbach, C.K. (1938): Clinical Studies of drug addiction. III *American Journal of Psychiatry,* **94**, 759–797.

Maggiolo, C. and Huidobro, F. (1961): Some features of the abstinence syndrome to morphine in mice, *Acta Physiol. Lat. Amer.* **11**, 201.

Martin, W.R. and Gorodetsky, C.W. (1965): Demonstration of tolerance to and physical dependence on N-allylnormorphine (nalorphine). *Journal of Pharmacology and experimental Therapeutics.* **150**, 437–442.

Martin, W.R., Eades, C.G., Thompson, W.O., Thompson, J.A., and Flanary, H.G., (1974): Morphine physical dependence in the dog. *Journal of Pharmacology and experimental Therapeutics.* **189**, 759–771.

Martin, W.R., Eades, C.G., Thompson, J.A., Huppler, R.E., and Gilbert, P.E. (1976): The effects of morphine and morphine-like drugs in the non-dependent and morphine-dependent chronic 'spinal' dog. *Journal of Pharmacology and experimental Therapeutics.* **197**, 517–532.

Swain, H.H., Villarreal, J.E. and Seevers, M.H. (1973): Personal communication as reported to the Committee on Problems of Drug Dependence, National Research Council, Addendum.

Swain, H.H., and Seevers, M.H. (1974): Personal communication as reported to the Committee on problems of Drug Dependence, National Research Council, Addendum.

Swain, H.H. and Seevers, M.H. (1975): Personal communication as reported to the Committee on Problems of Drug Dependence, National Research Council, Addendum.

Swain, H.H. and Seevers, M.H. (1976): Personal communication as reported to the Committee on Problems of Drug Dependence, National Research Council,

Teiger, D.G. (1974): Induction of physical dependence on morphine, codeine and meperidine in the rat by continuous infusion, *Journal of Pharmacology and experimental Therapeutics,* **190**, 408 – 415.

Teiger, D.G. (1976): Personal communication as reported to the Committee on Problems of Drug Dependence, National Research Council.

Villareal, J.E., and Seevers, M.H. (1967): Personal communication as reported to the Committee on Problems of Drug Dependence, National Research Council, Addendum 1.

Villarreal, J.E., and Seevers, M.H. (1968): Personal communication as reported to the Committee on Problems of Drug Dependence, National Research Council, Addendum 2.

Villarreal, J.E., and Seevers, M.H. (1968): Personal communication as reported to the Committee on Problems of Drug Dependence, National Research Council, Addendum 6.

Villarreal, J.E., and Karbowski, M.G. (1974): The actions of narcotic antagonists in morphine-dependent rhesus monkeys. *Narcotic Antagonists Advances in Biochemical Psychopharmacology* **8**, 273 – 290, Raven Press, New York.

Yanagita, T. (1973): An experimental framework for evaluation of dependence liability of various types of drugs in monkeys, *Bulletin of Narcotics,* **25**, 57–64.

## Discussion

*Session 4*

*Dr Potter.* Dr Bewley, have you any information about the circumstances in which dependence or drug abuse arose in your patients?

*Dr Bewley.* The majority are people who started using drugs for social reasons beginning with socially acceptable ones — tobacco, alcohol and moving on through cannabis and amphetamines to opiates and barbiturates with L.S.D. somewhere along the way. I also see a small number of people who have become dependent as a result of medical treatment, e.g. patients with haemophilia.

*Dr Fry.* Some patients fear the possibility of addiction more than post-operative pain. Are these patients more liable to develop dependence?

*Dr Bewley.* As regards the fear of addiction, I cannot really answer. I do not think there is any specific pre-addictive personality.

*Prof. Graham.* Have any other anaesthetists met this problem?

*Prof. Hobbs.* I have not met this in patients but I have in nurses. One has to give a certain degree of freedom to the nurses to decide when to give the post-operative analgesic, but because they seem to have been indoctrinated about the side effects and addictive effects they are reluctant to administer the drug in adequate amounts. As a result some patients may suffer unnecessarily.

*Prof. Campbell.* I agree our main problem is with the nursing staff, and this must be a reflection on our teaching.

*Dr West.* Quite often patients we admit from major hospitals have had no analgesic drug for many hours. Nurses are frightened to administer these analgesic drugs and doctors do not check that they have been given.

*Prof. Graham.* An analgesic which is long-acting may close this gap in practice.

*Prof. Joslin.* I favour passing the responsibility of requesting the analgesic to the patient. I find that patients in terminal care are extremely good at determining their analgesic requirements.

*Dr Geddes.* Another important aspect is that controlled drugs are locked away and at night there are often only junior nursing staff on the ward who do not have immediate access to the drugs. This can delay administration of the analgesics.

*Dr Rees-Jones.* Is there any new information on the use of *Beta* blocking drugs in the treatment of heroin addicts?

*Dr Lewis.* In our laboratories, Dr Alan Cowan was unable to confirm the results of the original animal studies.

*Dr Bewley.* People like Lars Gunne have endeavoured to replicate the original work and have also failed to do so.

*Prof. Dundee.* Will the relatively slow onset and long duration of action reduce the likelihood of abuse with buprenorphine?

*Dr Bewley.* I think that certain people will abuse any drug. There is a kind of hierarchy. Somebody who is dependent on opiates would prefer to have heroin than the longer acting drug, methadone.

*Mr Footerman.* Is there clinical evidence of tolerance to buprenorphine?

*Dr Robbie.* We have patients who have been on buprenorphine for weeks and months. Although there may be some evidence of mild tolerance, it has not been a problem. Further, even after months of usage we have had absolutely no problems of withdrawal.

*Dr Lewis.* We have results from Belgian studies of patients who, having been on buprenorphine for a long period, have been withdrawn, and given no further strong analgesic therapy. As far as I understand there has been no evidence of a withdrawal syndrome. Also following initial stabilisation, these patients have not required any increase in the dose of buprenorphine.

*Dr Rosen.* Could you clarify what is meant by onset and offset of action?

*Dr Lewis.* These terms refer to activity at the receptor site.

Buprenorphine is like methadone in being lipophilic and Professor Kosterlitz has shown how this results in a slow onset and an especially slow offset of effect, but unlike methadone, buprenorphine is a partial agonist.

These two factors may contribute to the lack of acute withdrawal symptoms on abrupt cessation of treatment or attempts to precipitate abstinence with antagonists.

*Dr Bewley*. Drugs have been introduced in the past as non-addictive and we have had to change our minds about them in due course. However, I think that we worry far too much about the small possibility of people becoming therapeutically dependent on opiates, and we tend to undertreat people.

# Session 5   Chairman: J. Parkhouse

Section 6    Chairman of Parkhouse

# 12. Management of the pain of myocardial infarction

J. R. HAMPTON

'I hope that when I die it will be by some relatively
painless process such as crucifixion'– from a letter
from a doctor who survived a myocardial infarction.

Myocardial infarction causes three sorts of problem: dysrhythmias, pump failure and
pain. The treatment of rhythm disorders has dominated the medical approach to
myocardial infarction in the past decade, and the management of dysrhythmias is
now relatively straightforward. The treatment of pump failure is relatively simple in
that mild degrees respond readily to conventional treatment with digitalis and diuretics,
while severe degrees of pump failure are essentially untreatable. It is pain that troubles
the patient most, and in this respect little progress has been made in the past quarter
of a century.

   The majority of patients are at home when they have their heart attack, and the
majority call for help from their general practitioners in the first instance (Hill and
Hampton,1976). Most patients have had their symptoms for about four hours by the
time medical aid is summoned (Fulton, Julian and Oliver,1969) and by then the major
risk of dysrhythmias is over. It has been shown that under such circumstances care
at home gives similar results to hospital care (Mather *et al*,1976; Hill, Hampton and
Mitchell,1977),so provided the general practitioner is confident that he can relieve
the patient's pain there is no need for hospital admission. At present, however, most
general practitioners believe that they should send all their patients with possible
heart attacks to hospital (Hampton, Morris and Mason,1975) and it may well be that
the lack of a good and safe analgesic weighs heavily in their attitude.

## Analgesics for myocardial infarction

The pain of a myocardial infarction can be intense, and it is often associated with
sweating and with vomiting. The patient is frightened. Even in the absence of
dysrhythmias his pulse is often rapid, although in the early stages excessive vagal
activity may induce a sinus bradycardia. The blood pressure is often low, although
in the presence of marked peripheral vasoconstriction (with or without left ventricular
failure) it may be elevated. Abnormalities of left ventricular performance may be
reflected by abnormal pressures in the right side of the heart, so the jugular venous
pressure may be raised, and if a catheter is inserted into the pulmonary artery, the
pressure there may be found to be high. Occasionally, however, despite the presence
of left ventricular failure the right sided pressures are low, and improve with volume
expansion.

Any analgesic that is to be used in a patient who may have such a complex and unpredictable haemodynamic state must itself be free of circulatory effects. Any analgesic that is to find widespread acceptance, particularly by the general practitioners who usually see the patient first, must have a low potential for abuse. Unfortunately the drugs with the greatest potency for pain relief and the least haemodynamic effects also have the highest abuse potential.

The best analgesic at present available for patients with myocardial infarction is diamorphine. In doses of 5 mg given intravenously or intramuscularly pain relief is rapid, the patient is sedated and his pain is replaced by a sensation that is usually described as pleasant. There are few, if any, untoward circulatory effects and there are definite advantages in the presence of left ventricular failure, for peripheral pooling of blood reduces pulmonary congestion. Vomiting is seldom a problem.

Morphine has a similar action to diamorphine, and frequently causes no haemodynamic changes at all (Lee *et al*,1976). On occasion, however, it causes severe bradycardia which requires treatment with atropine, and it may also induce hypotension. It has a less marked tranquillizing effect than diamorphine, and more often induces vomiting.

Because of the abuse potential, few general practitioners carry either diamorphine or morphine and restrict themselves to pethidine or pentazocine. Both of these drugs are less powerful analgesics than morphine, both may induce vomiting, and neither of them is a good tranquillizer. Pethidine usually induces little haemodynamic change other than occasional sinus tachycardia, but the effects of pentazocine are quite marked and are definitely undesirable. Pentazocine causes systemic and pulmonary vasoconstriction, so leading to a rise in systemic and pulmonary artery pressure (Jewitt, Maurer and Hubner, 1970). This leads to an increase in cardiac work, and so to an increase in myocardial oxygen demand. At the same time a negative inotropic effect causes a reduction in myocardial contractility. For these reasons pentazocine is contraindicated in patients with myocardial infarctions.

Less powerful analgesics than these four drugs are of little value, but one further agent has been found useful in the transport of patients to hospital. Entonox (Nitrous oxide 50 per cent and oxygen 50 per cent) can be administered by the patient himself, and is reasonably effective while having no significant haemodynamic consequences. Obviously the relatively cumbersome nature of an apparatus for gas administration restricts the use of this type of agent.

A general practitioner unwilling to carry diamorphine or morphine is therefore left with little choice other than pethidine, and there is clearly a need either for a new analgesic or for some alternative method of reducing pain. Before considering how this might be achieved we need to think about some of the characteristics of myocardial infarction pain.

### The nature of myocardial infarction pain

Myocardial infarction is one type of heart attack; this less specific term includes other clinical syndromes thought to be related to coronary artery disease, including sudden death and *angina pectoris.* Sudden death is the most dramatic form of heart attack, and although the patient may complain of pain, the major problem is dysrhythmia: by the very nature of the attack analgesia is not required. Myocardial infarction is properly speaking a pathological state involving ischaemic cardiac necrosis, which can only be recognised with certainty at necropsy. Its presence can, however, be inferred from the clinical picture, the electrocardiogram, and serum enzyme changes. *Angina pectoris* results from an imbalance between oxygen supply and demand in the myocardium. The pain is reversible and is not associated with structural changes in the heart, but apart from its duration angina pain is indistinguishable from that of myocardial infarction. This points to some very curious features of infarction pain.

The pain of myocardial infarction is variable and unpredictable, and its duration and intensity correlate very poorly with the apparent amount of heart muscle destruction. Indeed, myocardial infarction may be painless: up to 50 per cent of the old infarctions demonstrated at routine necropsy examinations have been claimed to be unrecognised in life, and in the Framingham study 11 per cent of patients who developed infarction patterns on their electrocardiograms during a period of observation had no chest pain at all.

If the origin of the pain of myocardial infarction is unclear, its precise mechanism is even more mysterious, for heart muscle behaves very differently from skeletal muscle. Infarction of a few cubic centimetres of skeletal muscle causes relatively little pain and almost no systemic disturbance. A myocardial infarction, on the other hand, may cause severe pain even though the actual mass of damaged muscle is small, and the systemic disturbance in terms of fever, malaise, and a rise in white blood cell count, erythrocyte sedimentation rate, and various serum enzymes can be dramatic. There are undoubtedly several differences between myocardial and skeletal muscle and in particular the two muscle types are microscopically different, the myocardial muscle fibres having a very much greater blood supply than those of skeletal muscle. Nothing, however, is known that satisfactorily explains the different effects of necrosis in the two muscle types.

The pain of myocardial infarction is curious in that it follows a different time course from the microscopical changes of infarction. Pain is usually the first symptom, and if the patient dies within a few hours of its onset there may be no microscopical changes to be found. Typically the pain lasts a few hours, and seldom as long as a day. The microscopical changes of myocardial fibre fragmentation and then degeneration with polymorph infiltration are not seen until several hours after the onset of pain, and are not really marked for as much as 24 hours.

Such observations, together with the similarity between the pain of angina and the pain of myocardial infarction, suggest that in infarction the pain arises not from muscle death but from ischaemia. Even if this is true, we do not know why ischaemic muscle is painful. Forty years ago Thomas Lewis showed that if forearm exercise was performed with a cuff around the upper arm inflated above systolic pressure, intense pain rapidly developed. This pain disappeared even more rapidly when the cuff was deflated, suggesting that a chemical substance was being washed out of the muscle. This 'pain substance' has never been positively identified, although there have been many suggestions as to its nature, including the accumulation of metabolic products, the activation of the kinin system, the production of prostaglandins, and so on. Whether such a 'pain substance' is produced by ischaemic heart muscle is unknown. A completely different explanation of myocardial pain is that it relates to a disorder of contraction like simple cramp rather than to any chemical abnormality.

Whatever the mechanism of ischaemic myocardial pain, it is an intriguing possibility that the pain of myocardial infarction might be helped by reducing ischaemia rather than by conventional analgesics.

## Possible mechanisms for reduction of myocardial ischaemia

Myocardial ischaemia occurs when myocardial oxygen demand exceeds supply. The oxygen supply to the heart depends on the arterial oxygen content and coronary blood flow; the latter is controlled by the calibre of the coronary arteries, by the diastolic blood pressure, and by the heart rate,which affects the diastolic period when most coronary flow occurs. The oxygen requirement of heart muscle depends on the heart rate, the ventricular wall tension (which parallels systolic blood pressure), the duration of systole and the contractile state of the heart. A reduction in heart rate should thus be beneficial,for it both improves coronary flow by prolonging the diastolic period, and reduces oxygen demand. A reduction in systolic pressure will reduce oxygen demand, but too great a reduction in diastolic pressure may reduce coronary flow.

Glyceryl trinitrate is effective in the treatment of angina because it reduces systolic pressure and the systolic pressure and heart rate product. It is ineffective in myocardial infarction possibly partly because of its transient effect, and partly because it induces a tachycardia. A reduction of both heart rate and systolic pressure can be induced by *Beta* blockade, and one would therefore predict that beta blockers would provide good pain relief in patients with myocardial infarction.

Such pain relief has been demonstrated with intravenous injections of metoprolol and practolol, the degree of pain relief correlating well with the reduction in heart rate, in systolic pressure, and in the product of heart rate and systolic pressure (Waagstein and Hjalmarson, 1975). Our own studies (unpublished data) have not, however, been so encouraging. We have found that patients given oral *Beta* blockers in maximum tolerated doses require as much 'conventional' analgesia as those given placebo '*Beta* blocker' tablets, and at present the prospects for control of cardiac pain by manipulation of the oxygen supply/demand relationship are not very encouraging.

## Buprenorphine and myocardial infarction

The drugs which are most effective in relieving the pain of a myocardial infarction and which have the least haemodynamic effects are diamorphine and morphine, but these are unpopular for use outside hospital because of their abuse potential. Pentazocine is unacceptable because of its haemodynamic effects, and pethidine is often not a sufficiently powerful analgesic agent. *Beta* blockers should relieve pain but do not appear very effective. There is clearly a need for a new powerful analgesic with low abuse potential, which has no undesirable haemodynamic effects; because buprenorphine appears in normal subjects and patients without cardiac problems to fulfil these requirements, we have made some preliminary studies of its effect on patients with myocardial infarction.

Of the first 15 patients treated with buprenorphine, ten were given diamorphine in the first instance and buprenorphine when their pain recurred; the other five received only buprenorphine as an analgesic. In each case pain relief was rapid, at most only mild discomfort remaining ten minutes after the intravenous injection of buprenorphine 0.3 mg. Thirteen patients became drowsy within a few minutes and were asleep within ten minutes, although they were easily aroused. Respiratory depression was not seen in any patient. The duration of pain relief varied, but appeared comparable to the effect of diamorphine 5 mg.

The only significant haemodynamic change observed was a mild fall in systemic (primarily systolic) blood pressure. Pulmonary artery pressures were measured by a fine polythene catheter inserted into a peripheral vein percutaneously and floated to the pulmonary artery, and Figure 12.1 shows a typical record. Injection of buprenorphine caused a small and transient fall in the pulmonary artery pressure; this

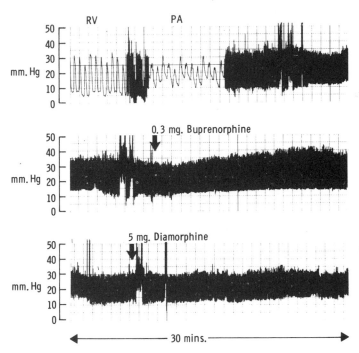

BUPRENORPHINE AND MYOCARDIAL INFARCTION

Fig. 12.1. Pulmonary artery pressure record from a patient with a myocardial infarction whose pain was treated with buprenorphine 0.3 mg. I.V., and four hours later with diamorphine 5 mg. I.V.

particular patient was given diamorphine when his pain recurred so that a comparison could be made, and it is clear that diamorphine had a very similar effect to buprenorphine. Figure 12.2 shows the changes observed in systemic and pulmonary pressure and in heart rate in five patients.

These preliminary studies suggest that in patients with myocardial infarction, buprenorphine 0.3 mg I.V. has approximately the same analgesic effect as diamorphine 5 mg. Buprenorphine, like diamorphine, seems to have no undesirable haemodynamic effects. Buprenorphine has proved popular with medical and nursing staff, and apparently with patients; further studies are in progress.

102

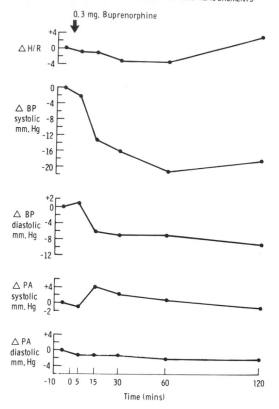

Fig. 12.2 Mean. changes in systemic and pulmonary blood pressure, and in heart rate, observed in 5 patients with myocardial infarctions whose pain was treated with buprenorphine 0.3 mg.

References

Fulton, M., Julian, D.G., Oliver, M.F. (1969) Sudden death and myocardial infarction. *Circulation,* **39**, Suppl. 4. Page 182.

Hampton, J.R., Morris, G.K., Mason, C. (1975). Survey of General Practitioners' attitudes to management of patients with heart attacks. *British Medical Journal,* **3**, 146.

Hill, J.D., and Hampton, J.R. (1976). Mode of referral to hospital of patients with heart attacks: relevance to home care and special ambulance services. *British Medical Journal,* **2**, 1035.

Hill, J.D., Hampton, J.R. and Mitchell, J.R.A. (1977). Randomised trial of home or hospital care for patients with heart attacks. In press.

Jewitt, D.E., Maurer, B.J., and Hubner, P.J.B. (1970) Increased pulmonary artery pressure after pentazocine in myocardial infarction. *British Medical Journal,* **1**, 795.

Lee, G., DeMaria, A.N., Amsterdam, E.A., Realyvasquez, P., Angel, J., Morrison, S., and Mason D.T. (1976) Comparative effects of morphine, meperidine and pentazocine on cardio-circulatory dynamics in patients with acute myocardial infarction. *American Journal of Medicine,* **60**, 949.

Mather, H.G., Morgan, D.C., Pearson, N.G., Read, K.L.Q., Shaw, D.B., Steed, G.R., Thorne, M.G., Lawrence, C.J., and Riley, J.S. (1976) Myocardial infarction: a comparison between home and hospital care for patients. *British Medical Journal,* **1**, 925.

Waagstein, F., and Hjalmarson, A.C. (1975) Double-blind study of the effect of cardioselective beta blockade on chest pain in acute myocardial infarction. *Acta Medica Scandinavica,* (Suppl.), 201.

# 13. The management of post-operative pain

D. CAMPBELL

The main practical problem in the effective management of post-operative pain is to ensure that the patient gets relief at the appropriate time. The techniques, with their relative advantages and disadvantages, are well known and there is a wide choice of drugs already available. While research continues to produce new compounds with fewer undesirable side effects, nevertheless I would submit that there is considerable room for improvement in the application of existing techniques and drugs, i.e. they could be more thoughtfully and efficiently applied, even in the absence of any further significant additions to our pharmaceutical armamentarium.

The crucial matter in most surgical wards is the staff/patient ratio, shortage of adequately trained nursing staff frequently vitiating the best-intentioned efforts of the medical staff. Even when this can be overcome there remains the subtle problem to which Parbrook and others have drawn our attention, the matter of the interplay of the patient's personality and his appreciation of pain and demand for its relief (Parbrook, Dalrymple & Steel,1973). The quiet stoic suffers considerable discomfort in silence while the vociferous neurotic will not tolerate even minimal pain and insistently demands its relief.

A recent post-operative study in Glasgow conducted by McNicol (1977) demonstrates how badly we sometimes do even in an apparently well-ordered institution.

A post-operative questionnaire (Fig. 13.1) shows the appalling results of simple lack of communication. A large number of patients, nearly 50 per cent, were

POST - OPERATIVE QUESTIONNAIRE (115 SURVEYED)

ARE YOU AWARE THAT YOUR ANAESTHETIST HAS PRESCRIBED PAIN KILLERS FOR YOU AND THAT ALL YOU HAVE TO DO IS ASK FOR THEM IF YOU NEED THEM?

| YES | NO |
|-----|-----|
| 60 | 55 |
| (52%) | (48%) |

Fig. 13.1.

apparently unaware that pain relief was readily accessible and in Figures 13.2 we see that patients often had to draw the attention of staff to the severity of their pain,

POST - OPERATIVE   QUESTIONNAIRE (115 SURVEYED)

HAVE YOU HAD CAUSE TO COMPLAIN ABOUT THE
SEVERITY OF YOUR PAIN AND ASK FOR SOMETHING
TO RELIEVE IT?

| YES | NO |
|---|---|
| 65 (56.5%) | 50 (43.5%) |

HAVING DONE SO, ARE YOU SATISFIED THAT YOU
WERE GIVEN SOMETHING TO RELIEVE YOUR PAIN AS
QUICKLY AS POSSIBLE?

| YES | NO |
|---|---|
| 54 (83% of | 11 |
| those who | |
| asked for | |
| analgesia) | |

Fig. 13.2.

requesting relief. Too seldom do the staff take the initiative in the process.

When attention was finally drawn to their plight, the majority of patients were satisfied with what was done for them but a fair number still suffered unrelieved discomfort.

There is little doubt that where staffing levels permit, the relief of post-operative pain is best managed by the intravenous administration of increments of the powerful narcotic analgesics. This technique, which is usually only practicable in post-operative recovery rooms and intensive care units, demands constant medical supervision. The parenteral therapy can be reinforced prior to painful procedures such as wound dressings and physiotherapy by self-administered inhalational analgesia. Outside of these special care areas, however, the problem remains. One attractive solution which is worthy of consideration is the routine administration immediately after surgery of an intramuscular dose of a long-acting analgesic. We are at present completing such a study comparing two doses of the long-acting analgesic, buprenorphine, with a standard dose of morphine in patients who have all undergone unilateral thoracotomy for pulmonary surgery.

The results from our initial pilot study, while in no way conclusive, suggest that $8 \mu g$/kilogram of buprenorphine can provide long term analgesia when given in this way more effectively than the standard 10 mg I.M. dose of morphine on demand, with a similar incidence of side effects. The lower $4 \mu g$/kg dose of buprenorphine would appear to be no more effective than morphine.

The patterns of pain relief provided by the two analgesics in the pilot study are demonstrated in Figure 13.3, when assessed on a lower pain scale.

Morphine gives an irregular pattern whereas buprenorphine, after a slower onset, provides more predictable and prolonged relief.

I would suggest that this technique, using buprenorphine or a similar long-acting analgesic, has a good deal to commend it for the relief of post-operative pain following major surgery.

There is still one area remaining where our efforts to relieve post-operative, or post-traumatic pain, are less than satisfactory.

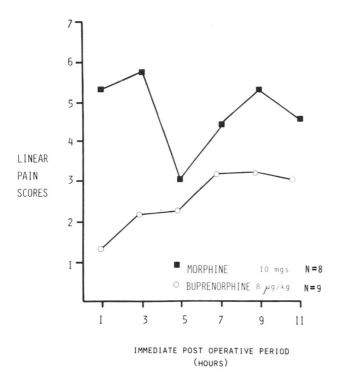

Fig. 13.3. Pattern of pain relief provided by intramuscular injection of morphine and buprenorphine.

About one-third of the patients treated in our busy Intensive Care Unit (approximately 150 per annum) require ventilator therapy for shorter or longer periods, many of these after extensive surgery or severe multiple injuries. The majority of these patients are unable to communicate with the nurse or doctor for much of the time and it is all too easy to assume that, as they lie immobilised by neuromuscular blockade, intermittently dosed with sedatives or analgesics, they suffer minimal distress or discomfort. That this is far from the case is all too frequently demonstrated by the spontaneous comments of patients who have successfully survived their injuries and our ministrations.

Two problems are involved, the first being the prevention of *awareness* in patients suffering little pain but on long periods of ventilator therapy and the second, the provision of adequate *analgesia.* Both, of course, may be indicated in any one patient. What is required is some form of monitoring which would reliably indicate when a patient was awake or in pain. Too often only 'the tell-tale tear' indicates belatedly that noxious stimuli are breaking through. Pain, as we are constantly being told, is largely a subjective phenomenon, but it has its autonomic components (Table 13.1) too, which might be capable of objective measurement.

All of these could be and have been used in attempts to monitor the patient's reaction to unpleasant stimuli, but none is of itself specific to this condition. Some years ago we

1. Heart rate

2. Systemic blood pressure

3. Central venous pressure

4. Skin and muscle blood flow

5. Skin resistance

6. Organ blood flow

Table 13.1. Autonomic response to pain.

attempted to apply a method of measuring changes in total forearm blood flow to this problem (Fig. 13.4), but the technique was abandoned because it was too clumsy and did not provide immediate 'on-line' information at the bedside (Telfer and Campbell, 1970).

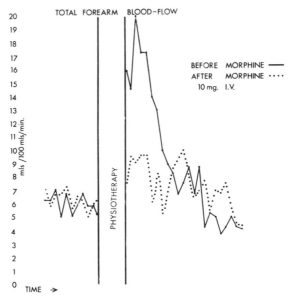

Fig. 13.4. Changes in total forearm blood flow in response to physiotherapy, and unpleasant stimulus.

All these patients are usually having cardiovascular measurements made at regular intervals, in some instances continuously, and observation of trends in response to stimulation, e.g. during tracheal suction or physiotherapy (Fig. 13.5) can be most informative to the observant clinician. The problem is more difficult in the less intensively monitored patients, though even here the astute clinician can make reasonable deductions from simpler measurements.

Changes in any *one* measurement may be unrelated to patient discomfort but

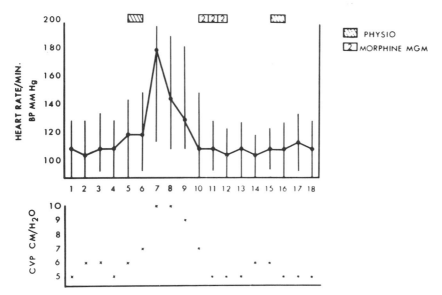

Fig. 13.5. Changes in heart rate, blood pressure and central venous pressure in response to physiotherapy.

when trends of *all* measurements are in the same direction then this is much more significant. We are at present trying to solve the problem in the latter patients by recording in parallel, changes in peripheral pulse (Fig. 13.6) both rate and amplitude, with changes in skin resistance, the psychogalvanic reflex (Figs. 13.7 and 13.8).

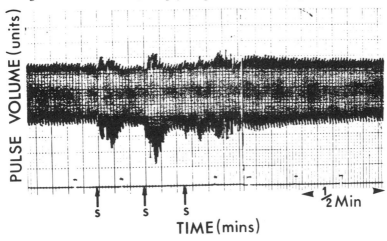

Fig. 13.6. Changes in peripheral pulse associated with patient discomfort.

The latter measurement, part of the well known lie-detector test, was tried and rejected by my late colleague, Walter Norris, in his earlier attempts to achieve objective measurement of sedation in premedicated patients prior to surgery (Nisbet, Norris and Brown, 1967). It is possible that in this new application it may have something more to offer.

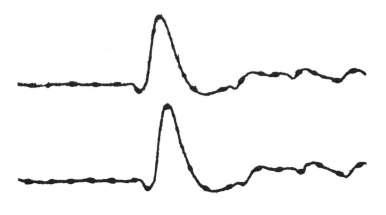

Fig. 13.7.

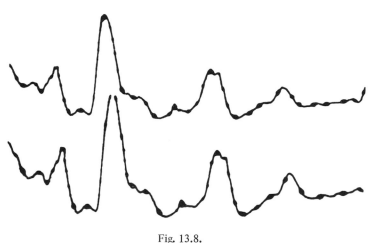

Fig. 13.8.

Fig. 13.7 and Fig. 13.8. Changes in skin resistance, the psycho-galvanic reflex associated with patient discomfort.

There is no easy answer to this fundamental problem of communication in Intensive Care Units, but its very nature should attract anaesthetists to the challenge and its eventual solution.

To conclude, it was Jacob Bigelow, the American physician, who wrote the epitaph for the memorial stone erected by the citizens of Boston, Massachusetts, to commemo. William Thomas Green Morton, the founder of anaesthesia, who died in 1868. These are the words he wrote:

'Inventor and Revealer of Anaesthetic Inhalation,
By whom pain in surgery was averted and annulled,

Before whom in all time surgery was agony,
Since whom *science has control of pain.'*

I am sure today we would accept that in our practice we fall short from time to time of this admirable standard, but I am equally sure that there is no worthier aim in the service of our patients.

## References

Nisbet, H.A., Norris, W., Brown, J. (1967): Objective Measurement of Sedation No.IV: The Measurement and Interpretation of Electrical Changes in the Skin. *British Journal of Anaesthesia.* **39**, 798.
McNicol, R.L. (1977): Personal communication.
Parbrook, G.D., Dalrymple, D.G., Steel, D.F. (1973): Personality Assessment of Post-operative Complications. *Journal of Psychosomatic Research.* **17**, 277.
Telfer, A.B.M., Campbell, D. (1970): Unpublished work.

# 14. The analgesic management of acute trauma

R. S. J. CLARKE

The best-known observations on trauma are probably those of Beecher, and I should admit at the outset that anyone who has been involved in an actual war, as he was, has probably seen far more casualties than we have in Belfast. Indeed a major hospital in the USA has a much larger intake resulting from deliberate violence than the Royal Victoria Hospital, Belfast.

## Beecher and the type of patient

When I was preparing this paper I looked through Beecher's *Resuscitation and Anesthe. for Wounded Men* (1949) and I was struck, first, by its continuing applicability, secondly, by the differences between military and civilian trauma and thirdly, by the changes in treatment which have occurred over 30 years. The first feature distinguishing the soldier is his initial fitness. He can tolerate severe injuries, massive blood loss and prolonged sepsis which would rapidly kill the unhealthy civilian. The other is his mental state and motivation. Beecher stresses that the wounded soldier is often euphoric and does not complain of pain as much as expected. He is released by the injury from fatigue, danger and fear of death and is quite pleased to find himself comfortably settled in a hospital.

The civilian casualty is rarely prepared for disaster. He is perhaps on his way home from a wedding when the car crashes, or he is blown up while drinking quietly in a pub. He cannot look at the injury with anything other than bitterness and needs not only analgesia but also tranquillization. However, unlike Beecher, I would make the point that the injured soldier needs much larger doses of analgesic than the civilian. He is often heavy and very strong and can accept 10 mg morphine intravenously like sterile water. A high proportion of traumatised civilians have taken a lot of alcohol. This is certainly an analgesic when administered intravenously (Dundee, J.W., 1970, unpublished studies) and clinically appears to reduce the dose of analgesic required. Of course, it often makes the patient aggressive and restless and in addition, it introduces the big problem of vomiting and soiling of the tracheobronchial tract. I shall not discuss this.

The time from injury on the streets of Belfast or indeed in most cities to surgical treatment is only a few minutes compared to the hours during World War II, and analgesia therefore need only be delayed briefly until a diagnosis is made, so that the total amount of suffering is reduced. The other advance is that emphasis on adequate fluid replacement has abolished thirst as the patient's most distressing complaint in traumatic shock (Beecher, 1949).


## Immediate care and pain relief

This subject has been excellently summarised by Baskett and Zorab (1975). They
define the duties of the medical man at the scene of an accident as:
1.  To preserve the life of the patient.
2.  To minimise complications due to injury.
3.  To reduce pain and suffering.
Leaving aside the first two problems, the necessity for early pain relief has long been
realised, but the frequency of disasters due to respiratory depression has discouraged
the effective use of strong analgesics. Entonox (50/50 nitrous oxide/oxygen from
one cylinder)therefore offers a great many advantages.
1.  It is rapidly effective.
2.  It has little effect on the cardiovascular and respiratory systems.
3.  It allows administration of 50 per cent oxygen and it has been shown that
    this results in much higher $PaO_2$ values than spontaneous respiration with
    an ordinary face mask (Baskett, Eltringham and Bennett, 1973).
4.  Its use encourages observation or assistance of ventilation.
5.  It can be administered by the patient.
The use of Entonox and other aids to resuscitation has been pioneered in the Bristol
area. It implies a unified ambulance administration and common medical policy so
that all seriously ill patients are channelled through a 'Mobile Resuscitation Unit'.
Ambulance personnel can then be trained in the use of Entonox as well as in general
resuscitation care. The use of this method of analgesia does not of course preclude
giving a stronger analgesic when there is someone competent to administer it, and at
least there are no serious interactions.

The most important aspects of analgesia are not what drugs to use but how to give
them, and the great advance advocated by Beecher, but still not fully learnt, has been
in giving opiates intravenously. This results in quicker and more reliable analgesia
and avoids the creation of a depot in poorly perfused tissue. Such a depot remains
ineffective and is perhaps even doubled or trebled by later medication, only to be
absorbed when the circulation improves hours later.

The need for analgesics varies greatly with the site of the lesion — abdominal
injuries and long bone fractures causing most pain while head and chest injuries
give least. In general, it is much more satisfactory if drugs can be withheld until the
surgical assessment has been made, though prolonged visits to the X-ray department
often necessitate not only analgesics, but also careful supervision. Delay is reasonable
if the patient can be got quickly into hospital but it is not really justifiable to leave
the patient to suffer. If the patient needs analgesics the main essential is to give the
drug intravenously and to send a note of the dose and time with him.

Special problems of interpretation exist in patients with head injuries. Not only
does the analgesic reduce the level of consciousness, but by constricting the pupils
it reduces the value of eye signs. In fact, however, patients with head injuries are the
least likely group to require analgesics, and treatment can usually be deferred. Similarly,
soft tissue injuries do not usually cause a lot of pain, and one of my earliest memories

of our present conflict is of seeing a man with a bullet (low velocity) in his gluteal region sleeping happily without surgery or analgesia. In some such patients tranquillizer may be of more value than analgesics.

### Analgesia and the intensive care unit

So far I have concentrated on the urgent aspects of analgesia but one of the great advances in treatment, in the United Kingdom at least, is the management of the traumatised patient in an intensive care unit. This means for instance that a patient with multiple rib fractures can be kept pain free, can have his respiratory function assessed and can be given physiotherapy several times a day. When there is no floating or flail segment of ribs and paradox is not excessive, good relief of pain often enables the patient to breathe and cough quite adequately. Certainly he will not keep his chest clear in the absence of adequate analgesia. The most useful method of providing controllable analgesia for such patients is the lignocaine infusion (e.g. 720 mg/500 ml 5% dextrose) 'piggy-backed' into the main drip and the rate controlled by the patient's response. Cardiologists have encountered convulsions with this mixture, but we believe that this complication is avoidable, or can be treated if necessary. The management of these patients, as with other forms of pain, is based on the principle that it is easier to keep a patient pain-free than to try to relieve pain when it occurs. Pain due to broken ribs is almost constant with each breath, and of course analgesia has also to ease the pain of coughing. Only for the additional stimulus of physiotherapy is a dose of intravenous narcotic required and if one is so fortunate as to have piped nitrous oxide, it is very useful for this purpose.

The other situation in the intensive care unit is the management of pain in the ventilated patient. The problem, of course, is the same whether the trauma is surgical or otherwise. Analgesia is easy when the respiration is suppressed by narcotics, since whatever opiate is used serves both functions. However, in patients who are paralysed the staff must make a positive effort to remember:

1. That the patient can hear.
2. That he may feel pain (Campbell, 1967).

Our only indications of distress to the patient are excessive sympathetic responses and it is probably best to keep up a basal level of sedative/analgesic therapy even if the patient has some impairment of consciousness. Our guide lines are to give the same type of analgesic regime to a paralysed patient as we would to a breathing patient — usually morphine and diazepam alternating every 2-3 hours. The dose is then increased if blood pressure or heart rate appear to indicate a reflex response to pain. The intravenous route is the most reliable route for the drugs but the rapid fluctuations in level need to be offset by frequent rather than high dosage. With diazepam there is also the special problem that the intramuscular route is painful and absorption is very erratic (McCaughey and Dundee, 1972), often leaving hard lumps in the tissues concerned.

Finally, I must mention the question of which analgesic to use, starting with the still popular pethidine. It is difficult to say that this drug has any real advantages (Eddy, Halbach and Braenden, 1957). It is of moderate duration, coming between the morphine group and the phenoperidine-fentanyl group. It is the most hypotensive of the opiates,due at least in part to histamine liberation. Phenoperidine is probably of shorter duration and less hypotensive in equipotent doses but there appears to be little advantage in using it for patients on a ventilator, unless ventilation is planned for a few hours only. The longer acting levorphanol and methadone would appear to be too cumulative for repeated administration every few hours. So, we return to morphine,which is still our drug of first choice.

## Summary

1.  The drug dosage should be adjusted to the patient's needs.
2.  The intravenous route should be used.
3.  Good documentation is essential.
4.  Opiates should be avoided in head injuries.
5.  Non-opiate analgesics should be used more frequently:
    a) Entonox
    b) Lignocaine infusion
6.  Diazepam should be given frequently as a tranquillizer, remembering that it enhances the respiratory depression of opiates.

### References

Baskett, P.J.F., Eltringham, R.J., and Bennett, J.A. (1973). An assessment of the oxygen tensions obtained with pre-mixed 50% nitrous oxide and oxygen mixture (Entonox) used for pain relief. *Anaesthesia, 28*, 449–450.

Baskett, P.J.F. and Zorab, J.S.M. (1975). Priorities in the immediate care of roadside and other traumatic casualties. *Anaesthesia, 30*, 80–87.

Beecher, H.K. (1949). *Resuscitation and anaesthesia for Wounded Men: The Management of Traumatic Shock.* Springfield, Illinois: C.C. Thomas.

Campbell, D. (1967). Pain relief in patients on ventilators. *British Journal of Anaesthesia, 39*, 736–742.

Eddy, N.B., Halbach, H. and Braenden, O.J. (1957). Synthetic substances with morphine-like effect. Clinical experience: potency, side effects, addiction liability. *Bulletin of the World Health Organisation, 17*, 569–863.

McCaughey, W. and Dundee, J.W. (1972). Comparison of the sedative effects of diazepam given by the oral and intramuscular routes. *British Journal of Anaesthesia, 44*, 901–902.

## Discussion

*Session 5*

*Prof. Kosterlitz.* Dr Clarke mentioned that injured soldiers required more morphine as premedication than would have been expected. This raises the question of whether endorphins are released during stress,and if so a situation of reduced sensitivity or partial tolerance to exogenous medication may be occurring.

*Dr Clarke.* I must admit that this was a clinical impression and we have no data on a body weight basis.

*Prof. Campbell.* I think we are comparing different groups of patients when the requirements of analgesic for the injured patient are compared with premedication for elective surgery.

*Prof. Parkhouse.* I feel this requires further investigation before conclusions can be drawn.

*Dr Fry.* Is muscle spasm a major cause of post-operative pain, and if so what treatment is recommended?

*Surgeon-Comm. Bertram.* Muscle spasm certainly plays a part in orthopaedic conditions and the use of diazepam together with mild analgesic alleviates the pain. I cannot comment on post-operative muscle spasm.

*Prof. Hobbs.* I do not see very much pain directly attributable to muscle spasm. We do see a lot of pain in patients following major surgery especially with thoraco-abdominal approaches. I would appreciate comments on our technique of hourly intravenous injections of small doses of morphine or omnopon.

*Prof. Campbell.* I think that Dr Rosen's method of self-administration of incremental doses could be used outside the field of obstetric pain and may be of great value clinically in view of the staffing problems which trouble us all.

More use might be made of regional techniques.

*Dr Rosen.* Of course, if patients are being ventilated one can use large doses of analgesic and these can be antagonised effectively with naloxone at the appropriate time.

*Prof. Campbell.* I agree, and by using a continuous infusion the patients may receive up to 10 mg morphine per hour. Althesin and/or diazepam are used for awareness, bearing in mind the problems of drug accumulation in patients under intensive care.

*Dr Lloyd.* Is thoracic epidural injection the treatment of choice in spontaneously breathing patients with crushed chest?

*Dr Clarke.* It may well be, but the technique is difficult and requires special expertise, and since many of the patients need ventilation because of respiratory impairment, analgesia is only one aspect.

*Prof. Hobbs.* Following on from this I would have thought the most important advance which could be achieved in the treatment of pain would be a drug with a long duration of action, which buprenorphine appears to have.

*Dr Robbie.* I agree, but in the worldwide context such drugs should have low abuse potential and this was the major reason why pentazocine had such an impetus, especially with the considerable percentage of people who are reluctant to handle strong narcotics.

*Prof. Hobbs.* Let us have both, but I still consider duration of action the most important when used in the controlled situation, and as we have heard any compound can be abused. Obviously, the lower the abuse potential so much the better, but if we were told that the abuse potential of buprenorphine was exactly the same as morphine it would still be preferable as a post-operative drug because of its length of action.

*Dr Clarke.* I would like to make a point regarding long duration of action. Although the effects of methadone last longer than six hours it is still prescribed on a 4—6 hourly basis which is often continued throughout the night. Patients are seen the following morning with respiratory rates of 4—6 per minute as a result of accumulation. It is thus vital that everyone using such a drug should be aware of its duration of action and the possibility of accumulation from too frequent administration.

*Prof. Dundee.* Would Dr Clarke like to comment on the use of Ketamine in pain associated with trauma?

*Dr Clarke.* I would not use it routinely but it is of value in intensive care patients requiring minor surgical procedures and who cannot be moved.

*Prof. Hobbs.* We have heard of the reluctance to use analgesics in adequate doses and that the fears associated with these agents are largely unfounded. How can we influence the attitudes of our medical and nursing students?

*Prof. Campbell.* I think the practical demonstration of drug action in man should begin for medical students in the second year in conjunction with the pharmacology curriculum. From this basis more meaningful teaching can be carried out in the clinical years. As the education of nurses is now largely out of our hands I cannot comment on the most appropriate time for training them on these important matters.

# Session 6    Chairman:  D. Robbie

# 15. Different approaches to the management of chronic pain

M. MEHTA

Since I am a very poor mathematician it is not surprising I could not even solve the simple puzzle which was set for my son in the old eleven plus examination:

4, 5, 6, 7, 8
61 52 63 94 ?

If you consider this in the conventional way you might start looking for the missing number in a series by calculating fractions and take a long time without arriving at the answer. However if you look at it as a child you will be seeing the problem in a different light and notice that the bottom numbers are squares of the uppers, but the figures are in reverse order. On this basis the correct answer is 46. This is lateral thinking, described by de Bono (1971) and Hannington-Kiff (1974), and is necessary for the management of many problems of chronic pain.

Acute pain seldom presents any difficulty because the diagnosis is known and treatment, directed at the cause, is invariably successful. Alternatively it may be only a question of tiding the patient over a difficult but well defined phase of his illness. In chronic pain this approach has limitations, because the aetiology is often uncertain or the cause apparent but irremovable, as in terminal cancer. In this symposium a great deal has been said about the measurement of pain and use of analgesic drugs, but this does not take into account the wide variety and advances in the treatment of pain by other means. In any case it is most inadvisable to confine therapy to one mode, however excellent this may be, and a review of current methods is available elsewhere (Mehta, 1973). Flexibility of approach is the key, and this is the reason why we no longer restrict ourselves to ablative procedures like cordotomy, or injection techniques like phenol chemical neurectomy in the spinal cord. Non-invasive methods like transcutaneous electric stimulation, acupuncture and hypnosis now come into the reckoning and are sometimes successful when more conventional therapy has been of no avail. Perhaps we ought to go even further and pay equal attention to prophylaxis, like the Chinese and others in the East. It might be profitable to train people at an early age to increase their tolerance to pain and severe discomfort by rigorous mental training, incorporating bio-feedback and possibly yoga or transcendental meditation.

It is a common misconception that only a particular hospital or specialist is competent to deal with problems of chronic pain. However, more than a high degree of individual expertise is required and de Bono rightly points out that an expert is like the man who digs a deep hole and the greater his knowledge the deeper the hole. Unfortunately there are occasions when the hole is so deep that the expert cannot look out and see if it has been started in the right place! A sense of proportion and realisation of the limitations of any technique are more likely when management lies in the hands of a group and is not decreed by any one person, however talented or versed in any particular skill. It is accepted that a multidisciplinary approach is necessary for diagnosis and treatment of all patients with pain of long standing. Many cases lie in a 'grey' area between the specialities and several different viewpoints may be necessary to achieve a satisfactory result. A great deal has been written about this multidisciplinary approach but in practice this principle cannot be interpreted too rigidly. It is extremely difficult for a group of busy specialists, involving possibly a neurologist, a neurosurgeon, a psychiatrist and an anaesthetist, to postpone heavy commitments elsewhere and find the time to meet regularly to discuss chronic pain patients. We prefer to do this informally and if necessary, admit the individual for a short hospital stay. This enables us to get several opinions without adhering to a strict timetable. Moreover, most patients are reluctant to face a committee, however erudite, if unknown to them. The consultant, to whom the patient is referred initially, initiates all investigations or referrals and integrates the information, communicating with the patient, his doctor and other members of the group.

Treatment also involves a great deal of flexibility and it is advantageous if the clinician extends his normal range of skills to include some which are unfamiliar. For example, as an anaesthetist I find it helpful to know the simpler aspects of psychotherapy, hypnosis and manipulation. This saves a great deal of time and unnecessary expertise. Where possible all difficult problems are dealt with by the member of the group best able to deal with them. The sole criterion for selection of treatment has to be the welfare of the patient but, even so, it is sometimes extremely difficult to discard a favourite technique, or one learned after a great deal of effort, in favour of another, which may be simple but available only in another department.

Finally, failure to relieve pain is no justification for projecting blame onto the patient and dismissing the symptoms as psychosomatic or imaginary. Sternback (1974) says 'Pain is whatever the patient says it is and exists wherever he says it does. Real, psychogenic or imaginary, however meaningless it may appear to the doctor, each patient is zealously convinced of the validity and importance of his pain.' It is well known that a small but significant number of patients will never admit to any improvement, even though there is demonstrable evidence, perhaps of sensory loss, to disprove this contention. Nevertheless, it is usually inadvisable to belittle an individual's complaints. Further investigation may reveal an organic basis or suggest a rational line of treatment. Alternatively, it will be necessary to seek help elsewhere.

These attitudes are illustrated by brief case histories from the author's practice. A young lady complained of continuing pain in the right iliac fossa and, because she was engaged to be married, was referred to a gynaecologist. Negative findings prompted the diagnosis of psychosomatic pain, but a simple nerve block completely relieved her symptoms even if this was only for a short time. Improvement was maintained by injections of 6 per cent aqueous phenol, and the syndrome is now recognised as nerve entrapment in the posterior wall of the rectus sheath (Mehta and Ranger, 1971).

Post-herpetic neuralgia in an elderly lady is often a very troublesome complaint, incompletely relieved by combinations of potent analgesic and anti-depressant drugs. Regional analgesia is also disappointing, so occasionally these patients are referred to a neurosurgeon, but even an extensive dorsal rhizotomy may not improve matters.

118

It is believed there is a retention loss of pain-inhibitory 'A' fibres in this condition and surgery accentuates the deficit. In this case we used a transcutaneous electric stimulator which raises a patient's pain threshold by recruitment of inhibitory pathways, and were able to keep her symptoms under control with considerably reduced amounts of simple analgesic drugs (Mehta, 1977).

Previous authors have mentioned the difficulties of measuring pain and, although this is essential for critical appraisal of new methods, it should not deter clinicians from using methods where the rationale is incompletely understood. After all if a patient has endured discomfort for a long period and is significantly relieved by any method for a reasonable length of time there cannot be any criticism of its use. A man's hand was badly injured in a traffic accident but excellently reconstituted by the plastic surgeon. Nevertheless continuing discomfort precluded his return to work. This was relieved by electric acupuncture. At the time I was unaware of the rationale behind this treatment but now, in the light of Professor Kosterlitz's paper, I suppose the improvement could be attributed to release of endorphin or related internal opiates.

My last case illustrates the virtues of a multidisciplinary approach. The X-ray appearance of a patient's lumbar vertebrae after extensive spinal fusion with a bone graft and several screws suggested a solid fusion and it was hard to imagine any movement. Nevertheless this patient continued to complain of severe mechanical-type low back pain with referred sciatica. My colleagues and I, in Norwich, believe that intervertebral disc protrusion has been over-emphasised in cases of this sort and we believed his pain emanated from stretching of the capsules of the facetal or posterior intervertebral joints, innervated by branches of the dorsal primary ramus. This hypothesis was confirmed by injection of local anaesthetic and subsequently relieved completely by diathermy with a radio-frequency probe (Mehta and Sluijter, 1977).

In this brief review, I have only been able to touch on the many ways of treating chronic pain. However, I hope I have emphasised what is more important, the necessity for a wider approach to the problems of pain and of placing consideration of the patient's welfare above all else.

### References

De Bono, E. (1971) — *The Use of Lateral Thinking,* England: Penguin, p.6.
Hannington-Kiff, J.G. (1974) — *Pain relief,* London: William Heinemann Books Ltd, p.158.
Mehta, M. (1973) — *Intractable Pain,* p.131, London and Toronto: W.B. Saunders Co Ltd.
Mehta, M. (1977) — The Principles of Pain, *Nursing Mirror,* **144**, 48.
Mehta, M. and Ranger, I. (1971) — Persistent Abdominal Wall Pain Treatment by Nerve Block, *Anaesthesia,* **26**, 330.
Mehta, M. and Sluijter, M.E. (1977) — A selective approach to percutaneous denervation in the lumbosacral area, *Communication to the Anglo-Dutch Pain Societies,* Leiden.
Sternback, R.A. (1974) — *Pain: Patients, Traits and Treatment,* New York: Academic Press, p.4.

# 16. Experiences in a pain relief unit 1970–1976

J. W. LLOYD

## Introduction

Pain is undoubtedly the worst taught, the least understood and the most neglected subject in medicine today. Perhaps for these reasons alone it has little difficulty in retaining its position as the most complex but certainly the most fascinating medical problem. It must be significant that opium ,which was first used in the third century B.C., is still, in 1977, the most commonly used analgesic.

In recent years some progress has been made, due in no small part to the gradual realisation that this is not a field for the occasional dabbler. Almost total involvement is necessary for any degree of success, and even then it is always hard earned.

There are, of course, still large gaps in our knowledge and these are being filled in by experience gained mostly in pain clinics, which are increasing in number throughout the country. Essentially outpatient clinics, they are excellent for initial assessment, diagnosis and prescription of analgesic drugs, but they do not generally have access to beds, a facility that I believe to be essential to the management of intractable pain.

## The role of a pain relief unit

There has been a Pain Clinic in Oxford since 1963 and in 1970 it graduated to a self-contained Pain Unit. It was the first of its kind in the National Health Service and some idea of the need for such Units must be gained from the fact that in the last two years more than 30 per cent of our work has come from outside the Area and the Region. The Unit has 10 beds and is situated on the site of a Community Hospital. It, therefore, has the advantage of providing immediate X-ray facilities, physiotherapy and a laboratory service. There is a large treatment room in the Unit which can be used for all standard procedures and also for minor day surgery. We feel that inclusion of day surgery in the Unit offers practical advantages for training anaesthetists in the use of local anaesthetic techniques.

Tables 16.1 and 16.2 show the number of admissions from 1970–1976 and the sources of referral of our patients.

We are, of course, concerned with the treatment of intractable pain, which has an inevitable, but misleading, association with cancer. When the Unit was opened, 75 per cent of our admissions were patients with cancer whereas today, seven years later, only 30 per cent of admissions are derived from this source. Unfortunately, this does

SCALE OF ATTENDANCES

| | 1970 Oct - Dec | 1971 | 1972 | 1973 | 1974 | 1975 | 1976 |
|---|---|---|---|---|---|---|---|
| Outpatients | 56 | 278 | 298 | 350 | 404 | 531 | 767 |
| Inpatients | 17 | 102 | 171 | 173 | 231 | 285 | 319 |

Table 16.1. Scale of attendances at the Oxford Pain Relief Unit 1970–1976.

| Source of Referral | |
|---|---|
| General Practitioner | 40% |
| Radiotherapist | 25% |
| Orthopaedic | 15% |
| Neurosurgical | 12% |
| Miscellaneous | 8% |

Table 16.2. Source of referral of patients to the Oxford Pain Relief Unit 1970–1976.

not mean that cancer is on the decline, but rather that the spectrum of admissions has widened. Certainly the pain of cancer is intractable but no more so than, for example, the low back pain of the young girl who has had three laminectomies, a spinal fusion, a de-roofing and is still incapacitated by pain. In our experience the treatment of cancer pain is far more successful than that of non-malignant conditions. Management of intractable pain presents a considerable problem, but we believe it is greatly simplified by the existence of a Pain Relief Unit. In the first instance the pressure on beds has been removed, so that we can accommodate patients for as long as necessary, with inevitable improvement in the standard of their assessment and over-all treatment. A multi-disciplinary approach can be practised; consultants from other specialties visit the patients on request and take part in a Combined Round to evaluate difficult cases every 10 days. These rounds are held after routine work and are regularly attended by a neurosurgeon, a radiotherapist, an orthopaedic surgeon and a physician. Terminal care can be provided if necessary.

Teaching and research form the basis of future medical practice, and in this respect a Pain Unit offers great potential. We have a full time research fellow attached to the Unit and in addition there is a rotational attachment of senior registrars for three days a week for three monthly periods, from the Nuffield Department of Anaesthetics.

## Experience in the Oxford Pain Unit, 1970 – 1976

Before the Unit opened in 1970, our main concern was to treat patients wherever they were and by whatever means were available. On occasions we modified existing techniques to advantage, but on no occasion could we lay claim to any original thought or advance. After 1970, and as a direct result of the Unit opening, the research facilities, and in particular the collection of data, were enormously improved. It therefore might be of interest to relate some of our work from that day until the present time.

In the first place, we needed to know the type of painful disorder to expect, and to have an estimate of the probable number to be admitted to the Unit each year. Cancer was a common reason for admission at that time and it can be seen (Table 16.3.) that, out of 244 patients admitted to the Unit with cancer, six sites of origin accounted for more than 70 per cent of the admissions.

INCIDENCE OF PAIN REFERRAL

| TYPES OF CARCINOMA | NO. ADMITTED FROM OCTOBER, 1970 TO OCTOBER, 1974. | O.R.H.A. NO. OF CASES REPORTED 1968 - 1972 | INCIDENCE PER 1000 CASES DIAGNOSED IN THE REGION. |
|---|---|---|---|
| LUNG | 67 | 5285 | 12.7 |
| BREAST | 46 | 3760 | 12.2 |
| CERVIX | 27 | 707 | 38.2 |
| RECTUM | 25 | 1515 | 16.5 |
| BLADDER | 23 | 1255 | 18.3 |
| PROSTATE | 15 | 1276 | 11.8 |
| PANCREAS | 13 | 942 | 13.8 |
| COLON | 12 | 2203 | 5.4 |
| STOMACH | 7 | 2069 | 3.4 |
| KIDNEYS | 5 | 421 | 11.9 |
| UTERUS | 3 | 670 | 4.5 |
| OVARY | 1 | 788 | 1.3 |

Table 16.3. Number of patients with cancer admitted to the Oxford Pain Relief Unit 1970–1974.

As the incidence of referral of these cases was in the order of 1 per cent and the total incidence of cancer in the Region was 7,500 cases a year we could predict that at least 75 patients with cancer would be admitted per year. In a literature search we were able to obtain comparative figures from only one paper, which came from Canada and quoted an incidence of referral of only 0.1 per cent. It is interesting to record that cancer of the cervix, which is relatively uncommon, is referred to the Unit more often than any other tumour. The incidence of pain referral per thousand cases is 38.2. If we now look at the percentage of cases surviving five years, we can see that cancer of the cervix is again the highest. (Table 16.4.). We are then left with the interesting speculation that here is a relatively uncommon tumour associated with a

| TYPE OF CARCINOMA TREATED AT PAIN RELIEF UNIT | O.R.H.A. NO. OF CASES REPORTED 1967 | FIVE YEAR SURVIVAL |
|---|---|---|
| LUNG | 985 | 6.4 |
| BREAST | 267 | 29.6 |
| CERVIX | 126 | 59.5 |
| RECTUM | 307 | 23.8 |
| BLADDER | 245 | 34.3 |
| PROSTATE | 244 | 15.6 |
| PANCREAS | 155 | 1.9 |
| COLON | 461 | 16.1 |
| STOMACH | 404 | 4.2 |
| KIDNEY | 80 | 21.3 |
| UTERUS | 124 | 51.6 |
| OVARY | 177 | 16.9 |

Table 16.4. Percentage five-year survival of patients referred to the Oxford Pain Relief Unit.

high incidence of pain and also having a high five year survival rate.

Next, we attempted to show how patients reported their pain. Pain is essentially a subjective phenomenon and therefore the patient's own assessment of severity throughout the day was recorded. 54 patients, all suffering from intractable pain, indicated the intensity of their pain on a visual analogue scale every two hours from 8.00 a.m. to 10.00 p.m. on seven successive days.

41 patients provided complete reports, from which we were able to demonstrate a diurnal (over 12 hours) variation of pain intensity reaching a maximum at 10 p.m., the time of the last assessment. (Figs. 16.1 and 16.2).

Comparing the diurnal variation of pain in patients who went out to work and those who stayed at home, it can be seen that in the latter group there is a significant increase in reported pain (Fig. 16.3). It would appear that, from the practical aspect alone, patients may need different amounts of analgesics at different times of the day. Where possible, it would seem beneficial to indulge in activity to get them out of the house and to anticipate their peaks of pain by prescription of analgesics.

Another study concerned factors which may be related to the degree of pain reported by patients. Both acidosis (Lindahl, 1974) and alkalosis (Evans, 1972) have

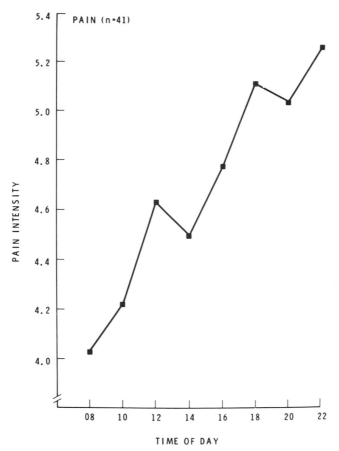

Fig. 16.1. Diurnal variation of pain intensity.

been described in association with intractable pain. In our series of 52 patients pH was normal, but hyperventilation and low $PCO_2$ were consistent findings.

The radial artery was cannulated in all 52 patients admitted to the Unit and $PaCO_2$, $PCO_2$ and pH were measured every two hours, for periods ranging from 12 to 24 hours. Treatment of pain resulted in relief for 30 patients, 10 of whom were available for follow-up of blood gas estimations. The results in Table 16.5 showed that they all had a low pre-treatment $PCO_2$ and normal pH. After relief of pain there was a statistically significant rise in $PCO_2$ without a fall in pH. These findings show that intractable pain was accompanied by hyperventilation and that relief of pain produced a decrease in ventilation. It would, therefore, seem reasonable to assume that if hyperventilation was abolished by pain relief, pain itself was the cause of that hyperventilation. It is also tempting to suggest that patients with chronic pain should all have a low $PCO_2$, which may provide an objective measurement of pain.

Finally, in considering treatment it is always worth remembering that technical expertise, however valuable, is of minor importance compared with a proper under-standing of the patient. Standard methods of pain relief usually involve the interrup-tion of pain pathways or the prescription of analgesic drugs. Many of these methods

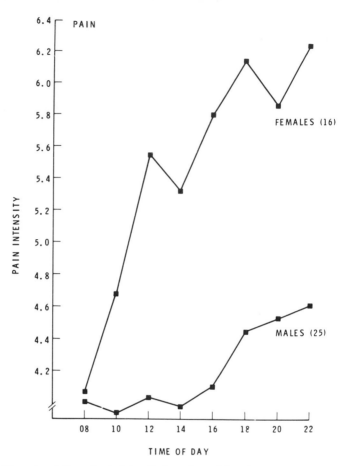

Fig. 16.2. Diurnal variation of pain intensity in males and females.

PaCO$_2$ and pH following Pain Relief

| No. | Sex | Age | Pre-treatment PaCO$_2$ | Post-treatment PaCO$_2$ | Pre-treatment pH** | Post-treatment pH | Group | Treatment |
|---|---|---|---|---|---|---|---|---|
| 5 | F | 56 | 34.5 | 35.9 | | 7.46 | Back | Spinothalmic cordotomy |
| 6* | F | 33 | 26.7 | 33.8 | 7.43 | 7.42 | Back | Iced cold normal saline CSF replacement |
| 11* | M | 49 | 32.2 | 36.0 | 7.40 | 7.41 | Back | Extradural injection of local anaesthetic + steroid |
| 12* | F | 22 | 29.8 | 34.4 | 7.43 | 7.38 | Back | Iced cold normal saline CSF replacement |
| 18 | M | 64 | 29.4 | 36.8 | 7.41 | 7.40 | Cancer | Intrathecal chlorocresol |
| 24 | M | 60 | 30.1 | 36.1 | 7.42 | 7.43 | Cancer | Intrathecal chlorocresol |
| 27 | F | 34 | 33.2 | 37.3 | 7.44 | 7.43 | Cancer | Intrathecal phenol 5% |
| 28 | F | 79 | 31.4 | 37.6 | 7.41 | 7.42 | Cancer | Intrathecal phenol 5% |
| 31 | F | 73 | 34.1 | 38.2 | 7.45 | 7.44 | Cancer | CSF barbotage |
| 32 | M | 57 | 30.9 | 37.4 | 7.43 | 7.41 | Cancer | Intercostal nerve block cryoprobe |

* single blood-gas estimations
** the absent result is due to a technical fault

Table 16.5. The effect of pain relief on PaCO$_2$ and pH in patients admitted to a pain relief unit.

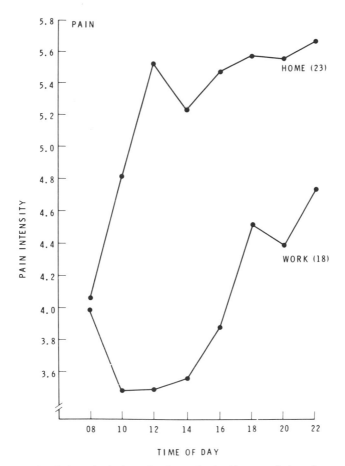

Fig. 16.3. Diurnal variation of pain intensity for patients at home and at work.

are now well-established, but that is surely no reason for complacency.

Following the work of Hitchcock (1967) in irrigating the cerebrospinal fluid (csf) with hypothermic saline we feel that it was a logical sequel to use the patient's own c.s.f. We therefore introduced barbotage, which consists of the alternate withdrawal of 20 mls of c.s.f. to and from the subarachnoid space. In 50 patients, 35 obtained relief lasting from three days to seven months. We are still unsure of the mechanism of relief, but believe that it is probably due to pressure effect causing local cord asphyxia.

In 1976, following the work of Baron Larre in 1812, we introduced cryoanalgesia. The development of a small needle probe with a built-in thermocouple and stimulator at the tip enables a nerve to be located blindly.

Using the well-known Amoils (1965) principle (Fig. 16.4) an ice ball is then generated at the tip of the probe to encompass the nerve. The temperature at the centre of the ice ball is minus 70°C. This technique gives a predictable and reversible conduction block of between 15–25 days and in some patients relief has lasted for

## JOULE – THOMPSON PRINCIPLE

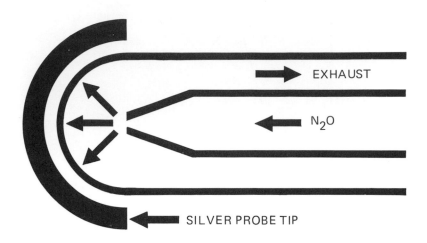

EXHAUST

$N_2O$

SILVER PROBE TIP

AMOILS S.P. (1967) THE JOULE THOMPSON
CRYOPROBE
ARCH. OPHTHAL. 78,201

Fig. 16.4.

up to 160 days with early recovery of motor and sensory function. Treatment of the
facial neuralgias has been particularly encouraging (Tables 16.6 and 16.7). It can be
seen that in this case the median duration of pain relief was 116 days, decidedly
longer than from section of the nerve.

| Diagnosis | |
|---|---|
| Post Herpetic Neuralgia | 9 |
| Neuralgia of Unknown Aetiology (Atypical Facial Neuralgia, Tic Doloureux | 8 |
| Post Surgical Neuralgia | 3 |
| Malignant Disease | 1 |
| Total | 21 |

Table 16.6. Types of neuralgia treated by cryoanalgesia.

| | Cryoanalgesia | Freeze and Section |
|---|---|---|
| **Pain Relief** | Days | Days |
| Median duration | 116 | 38 |
| Range | 0 – 257 | 0 – 84 |
| **Sensory Loss** | | |
| Median duration | 49 | 131 |
| Range | 4 – 117 | 21 – 339 |

Table 16.7. Duration of pain relief in patients with facial neuralgia treated by cryoanalgesia or nerve section.

### References

Amoils, S.P. (1965) *Archives of Ophthalmology*, 78, 201.

Evans, R.J., (1972) Acid-base changes in patients with intractable pain and malignancy, *Canadian Journal of Surgery*, 15, 37.

Hitchcock, E.R., (1967) Hypothermic subarachnoid irrigation for intractable pain, *Lancet*, 1, 1133.

Larre, D.J., (1812) *Surgical memoirs of campaigns of Russia, Germany and France.* Translated by Mercer, J.C., Philadelphia: Carey & Lea. p. 293.

Lindahl, O. (1974) Pain – a general chemical explanation. *Advances in Neurology*, 4, Ed. J.J. Bonica, New York, Raven Press, p.p. 45 – 47.

### Discussion

*Session 6A.*

*Dr Alexander.* Can Dr Lloyd tell us how applicable is cryoanalgesia to mixed nerves?

*Dr Lloyd.* We have restricted its use to nerves with little motor function. In one case freezing the first lumbar paravertebral nerve for stump pain gave complete relief. However, motor function returned within 24 hours while sensory loss and pain relief persisted for 14 days.

Our observations contradict the original work by Denny Brown, who found that pain fibres were the most resistant to temperature, admittedly only down to –4°C.

We would prefer to freeze only the sensory dorsal ganglion, but this must be very difficult because of the close proximity of the motor root.

*Dr Raftery.* Can Dr Mehta comment on the differential diagnosis of low back pain and on the use of differential local anaesthetic block in deciding the exact derivation of the pain?

*Dr Mehta.* We use an epidural catheter and local anaesthetic to differentiate between organic pain, assumed pain and that with a marked psychological overlay. However, this has not been of great value in differentiating between pain due to central disc protrusion and that caused by lateral or mechanical type of pain.

Following the introduction of facet rhizotomy by Skyrme-Rees, which we thought totally unselective, we decided to use local anaesthetic with radio-opaque dye at the point where the dorsal primary ramus passes through the intertransverse ligament. This enables us to decide whether this is the source of pain. We then use the radio-frequency probe at the level where pain relief is complete.

*Dr Raftery.* My impression is that the incidence of carcinoma of the cervix is falling. Is this due to improved use of cytotoxic drugs or improved early diagnosis?

*Dr Alexander.* I would think this is a problem of referral and that patients are only transferred when they have a real pain problem, or are problem patients or have problem relatives.

*Dr Burn.* May I congratulate Dr Lloyd on his papers? However, I disagree that beds are necessary for clinicians who are treating pain. Is it not better to treat such patients in the beds of their primary physician so that all aspects of therapy can continue?

*Dr Lloyd.* I feel that the patients benefit from being in a central point where they feel they are receiving all the attention they would like. Added to this we undertake a combined round which includes a radiotherapist and a neurosurgeon. Further, if we do not have our own beds the pressure on beds in other departments makes it almost impossible to admit patients for specific procedures.

*Dr West.* The answer to this may be in the use of the 'symptom control team' as in St Lukes, New York and now being established at St Thomas's. The team of doctors, nurses, social workers and chaplain are called to wherever the patient is situated to give advice and specialist therapy as appropriate.

*Dr Rosen.* I feel it is clear that anaesthetists should be involved in this area. However, before advocating such wide usage of such teams we should have the results of carefully controlled studies which will identify their value.

Dr Lloyd has started this process with the data he presented but we still do not know how many patients are not referred.

*Dr Lloyd.* Initially, 75 per cent of our patients had cancer, now we find more and more referral of non-malignant patients and eventually we will have figures on this group from which a base-line can be decided and from which future requirements may be visualised.

*Dr Mehta.* A great deal of information on this aspect is being collected on an international basis by Dr Haydn Dyer in Western Australia and the data have been forwarded to me.

The major drawback to date in regard to accumulation of hard data has been the fact that most anaesthetists interested in this field have not been allocated sessions for the specific purpose. I would suggest that until we have more pain relief units the facts and figures will remain difficult to obtain.

# 17. Doctors and the dying patient

E. WILKES

In a sociological survey of 71 different cultures spread inevitably over many parts of the world, five aspirations seemed common to all. Since life is sweet the first aspiration was to live for a long time, but the second was to retain one's faculties, preserving one's waning strength and gradually being able to relax from the burdens of the day. One wanted, however, at the same time to have the rights and respect proper for a senior member of society. This implies the retaining of some suitable active role in community activities,and the final, and perhaps most crucial, aspiration was to have a timely death which was honourable and dignified and which, with some cultures, could carry important implications for a life hereafter.

Against these very reasonable aspirations, how does our industrial and mobile society measure up? Let us take these points one at a time.

Life is indeed sweet and it is good to live a long time: but the tremendous expansion of the life-expectancy over the last half-century has carried with it heavy burdens for patients, for families, and for society at large. This is because it is not always possible to retain one's faculties and indeed there are obvious parallels, as life closes, with the dangers of life's beginning. The baby can be born on time, or as a premature or post-mature baby, and there are different properties and hazards associated with these. It is a tragedy also to die prematurely of some sudden cardiac catastrophe in one's forties and at the height of one's powers. A more frequent problem is to live too long, to have, as it were, a post-mature death, so that one's body has survived long after one's capacity to be independent, inquisitive, even mobile.

Although the deterioration of intellectual faculties is perhaps the most distressing and the problem on the largest scale, the physical wear and tear of a prolonged life-span creates more demand for the expensive and burdensome management of renal failure, or for a massive programme of replacement arthroplasties, which would be unattainable even without major economic problems. This is an area of high-technology medicine, and one in which medical historians of the late 20th century can take pride.

In a society, however, dedicated to the ruthless advances of technology it is very difficult to preserve the rights or respect formerly due to the old, or for a positive active role to be retained by those whose expertise belongs to a bygone age of 10, 20 or even 50 years before. The old are therefore tremendously devalued in a world which cannot use their talents and which may in fact pass their talents by for years before their formal retirement. The burden on the younger members of the family is accepted dutifully over many years, but is only rarely and atypically a matter for pleasure. It is one of the more grinding and dreary sacrifices of middle-age and our society has lost pleasure and instruction from the company of the old.

The story does not alter in its sadness when one looks at the way we deal with that crucial need for a timely, honourable and dignified end. The big killers in our society are heart disease, cancer and stroke.

Heart disease can cloud the final years with increasing pain and ever encroaching restriction of physical resources. Patients adjust well to this on the whole, and have less of the fear so typical of the patient dying slowly from malignant disease. There is to some degree justification for this improved morale, since they are likely to be bedfast or incontinent for a shorter period of time than those suffering from disseminated cancer, and their pain is likely to be less prolonged and less severe in the great majority of cases.

The management of stroke is still somewhat neglected. Disturbances of speech are reasonably common and high quality corrective speech therapy only available in comparatively few centres. The mobilisation after a stroke is of course very effective in well-staffed units with specialised experience and enthusiasm. Again, however, these units are not uniformly available, and even when they do exist and achieve a most satisfactory degree of rehabilitation, there is a tremendous gap between the rehabilitation resources of the in-patient and the perfunctory and under-resourced care available in the community. Many patients who have attained a temporary and spurious independence in the hospital department of occupational therapy lose this in the less conveniently designed bathrooms and kitchens of their own homes. They therefore live in a no-man's land, neglected and deteriorating at home, or living in the non-world of hospital, holding their own with some difficulty, but gradually overwhelmed by the processes of institutionalisation.

However, it is in the field of malignant disease that most work has been done and most interest taken, since here we enter the world of fear and suffering, treated so often by an uneasy compounding of drugs, silence and false reassurance.

In a survey of Sheffield general practitioners only 13 per cent of dying patients had their situation frankly discussed with their family doctor (Ward, 1974): yet the general practitioners thought that up to 50 per cent of their patients knew that they were dying. These figures, as one can perhaps expect, are somewhat lower than hospital survey figures, which tend to show a somewhat higher proportion of terminal patients with a full recognition of their real predicament (Hinton, 1967). My view is that all these figures will perpetually be changing, since our patients wish to know more and more about the true facts of their illness and to be involved more and more in the management of their case.

Paradoxically, therefore, it may well be the senior and more experienced clinicians who are most out of touch with the needs of their patients and the more junior doctors who exhibit a more sensitive understanding. Younger patients, especially, require to be involved in discussions about any possible options open to them and may insist on being told of the incurable nature of their ailment. This can lead to a heavy and demanding burden of counselling and support over many months, but is nonetheless a duty for which time and skill and patience must be found.

In a survey of the common sites of cancer, it was found that the natural history of primary growths of lung, breast, genital or gastrointestinal tracts differed comparative little in the pattern of terminal disease. Of those dying at home, only some 15 per cent needed detailed nursing care for longer than six weeks, 50 per cent had no important pain, and again only 12 per cent needed a higher quality of care than was available in their own home (Wilkes 1965).

We have paid lip-service ceaselessly to the ideal of dying in one's own home. This is partly a folk-tradition, since the home is a place to die in as well as to live in, and something like 95 per cent of deaths in the last century occurred at home. One must, I think, confess that a major factor buttressing the willingness of patients to die nowhere but in their own home, where this is possible, is an increasing mistrust as to the quality of care they will receive in the hospitals. They will be living in a ward as devoid of privacy as any stable; they will be living in a world where a fairly strict régime is essential to permit the survival of the harassed and understaffed nurses; whilst the quality of food, of medication, even of manners is variable, and known to be so. No ill person can deal adequately with strangers, and yet, when one has said all that, why is it that the proportion of deaths occurring in the hospitals is increasing each year and that, despite obvious regional variations, only about one third of deaths are now occurring at home? To die in hospital, however unwillingly, is now the norm and the factors that produce this are the expensive and cramped housing, the part-time or the full-time job, which makes the full-time mother-housekeeper more the exception than the rule, and most of all, the increasing age of our society, such that in one survey it was found that no less than 15 per cent of cancer patients dying at home were being cared for by relatives who were themselves over 70 years of age (Wilkes, 1965).

We have therefore elaborated a routine in which a terminal illness presents to the general practitioner and is usually referred for further investigation, and perhaps for surgery, to the local hospital. Follow-up is maintained at a variable interval, and although many patients are discharged to purely general practitioner follow-up, many others keep attending the out-patients over the years until in time they have to be re-admitted for their last few days.

What perhaps does need emphasis is the degree to which patients are admitted to die among strangers (Ward, 1974). Most patients who die in hospital will have had most of their care in their last month on earth given to them by relatives at home, and terminal admissions average on the whole something like two weeks in duration. Some, of course, will need institutionalisation for months before death, but these are a small minority. A bigger minority are those who die within hours of admission, causing perhaps a good deal of guilt and regret on the part of the spouse and making up in one hospice series something like 10 per cent of the total admissions (Wilkes, 1974). The teaching hospitals have not shown a major pre-occupation with this area of medicine and admit only some 2 per cent of the deaths of the United Kingdom (Cartwright, Hockey and Anderson, 1973).

The primary site naturally has some impact on the problems needing high-quality nursing care. Although the bronchial carcinoma is likely to be easily the most frequent tumour needing admission, such cases tend to have a much shorter prognosis than the breast cancers. These latter take, in the experience of one terminal care unit, on average no less than two and a half times the bed-days per year that are required for the greater number of primary lung tumours (Wilkes, 1974).

Neoplasms of the lower genital tract, especially in the female, are likely to give rise to fistulae. Confusion can be a most demoralising symptom to deal with at home, and incontinence can prove, with the additional laundry and the shame and guilt of the patient, a major indication for admission to hospital.

The commonest of all problems, however, in cases dying from disseminated malignant disease, is pain. This symptom was present to a dominant degree in 58 per cent of a series of admissions admitted to a unit specialising in the terminally ill. It is important that adequate pain control should be directed towards the patient and not towards the pain. To help the patients adjust to their situation, to participate in a controlled way with their grief for the loss of the person they used to be, and to fill their day in with some form of companionship or occupation which gives them pleasure or which they feel to be of value, these can be of as much help in pain control as the latest or most important analgesic drug. One of the great potentiators of pain, however, is a feeling of isolation, of an inability to communicate with the doctors, who tend to wear white coats and to go round in small flocks like supercilious sheep, and who can only rarely and atypically be persuaded to sit on the bed and to talk patiently and frankly about the problems the patient is facing among all the expensive clutter and the teamwork of modern medicine and yet, so often, heartbreakingly alone.

Doctors of course are not exempt from that inexperience and uncertainty with which dying patients are encountered in our society. As medical students, hardly any of them have seen anyone die or had personal experience of bereavement. They acquire an armour during their years of clinical apprenticeship and they are able to cope with most of the challenges that present to them more than adequately. Their vulnerability, however, can sometimes be most obvious when they are dealing with the terminally ill. Doctors who have direct clinical contact with patients have been shown to have a higher incidence of alcoholism, psychiatric consultation, or marital breakdown than those of similar socio-economic status, or other doctors who do not have direct clinical responsibility (Vaillant, Sobowale and McArthur, 1972). Many of them have not the technique to share problems with the patient speedily and to acquire relationships in depth in a matter of minutes. This is by no means a routine part of their professional training. When they are faced with a dying patient they are tempted to sacrifice the unexpressed needs of the patient to their own peace of mind. The problems of the doctor do not end even here.

Despite the decades of progress the management of malignant disease is to some degree an area of opinion rather than of fact, and when the routine modalities of treatment have been exhausted and the patient has not responded satisfactorily, then the therapeutic regime advised by the doctor becomes more and more a personal choice among the restricted options available. Those who have a genuine oncological enthusiasm and training will therefore, to an increasing degree, be giving incurably ill patients nausea, vomiting, alopecia and marrow depression, in what may be an answer to the doctor's problems rather than the patient's. They may be finding a role in treating patients who would relish, in the few precious weeks left to them, liberation from potent and expensive cytotoxic drugs.

Most cytotoxic drugs given to patients in our hospitals today are given for somewhat ill-thought-out reasons and may indeed be making the burden of illness heavier rather than lighter. The distress of the relatives must also be weighed in the balance together with the distress of the patient, when one is assessing how justifiable the cytotoxic regimes are in certain cases.

One must not be too flabby or obscurantist about this. It is fatuous and poor medicine to pour cytotoxic drugs into patients who have only a few weeks to live. It would be equally improper to resent the transient, if burdensome, side effects for patients whose Hodgkins disease or whose leukaemia has a quite different outlook today as a consequence of the aggressive and expensive therapy of recent years, so successful in this restricted field.

It is not an easy time in which to care for the incurably ill. One is walking a perpetual therapeutic tightrope between unjustifiable neglect and naive and ill-founded enthusiasm. In this situation experience, humanity, and a genuine knowledge of the limitations and potential of the various modalities of treatment, are as essential as a capacity to share the fears and burdens of the patient. In an economically stringent situation, with a high work-load, with staff of variable quality, it may be justifiable on occasion to cast a look of envy at those who work in special units geared to the terminally ill and who have fought for, and gained, increasing acceptance in the changing world of modern medicine.

### References

Cartwright, A., Hockey, L., Anderson, J.L. (1973): *Life Before Death,* Routledge and Kegan Paul.
Hinton, J.M. (1967) *Dying,* England: Penguin.
Vaillant, G.E., Sobowale, N.C., and McArthur, C.(1972): Some psychologic vulnerabilities of physicians. *New England Journal of Medicine.* **287**, 372–375.
Ward, A.W. (1974): Terminal care in malignant disease. *Social Sciences and Medicine.* 8, 413.
Wilkes, E. (1965): Terminal cancer at home. *Lancet,* 1, 799.
Wilkes, E. (1974): Michael Williams Lecture: Some problems in cancer management. *Proceedings of the Royal Society of Medicine,* 67, 1001–1008.

# 18. The role of residential care in terminal illness

F. R. GUSTERSON

I still have a copy of the pharmacopoeia of my old hospital, dated 1931, which was acquired when I set out to practise my skill on an unsuspecting public. All the drugs known to us at that time are listed in this slender volume, the only analgesics and sedatives being acetanilidine, acetylsalicylic acid, barbitone and its sodium salt, two strengths of opium, ½ and 1 grain, and one twelfth of a grain of diamorphine. In those days when the latter was regarded as a useful ingredient of cough linctus, we wrote our prescriptions with meticulous care, always starting with the sign R for 'recipe' which means 'take thou'. A small cross was then added to the tail of the $R_X$ as an invocation to the gods, 'and may it do him some good'. In view of Professor Wilkes's comments about cytotoxic agents, this custom should be continued, but with a modified interpretation, 'I hope it does him no harm'.

The strong analgesic of choice in our special care unit is a simple solution of diamorphine starting with a dose of 2.5 mg in 10 ml water. This has the advantage that the dose of diamorphine can be titrated according to the requirements of individual patients without any apparent change in the volume of successive doses. We step up the dose of diamorphine to 20 mg if necessary, but still in 10 ml of water. Cocaine is not included in our mixture and we find that, used in this way, diamorphine can be stopped very quickly without problems of addiction should relief of pain no longer be necessary. A patient must be mentally alert as well as free of pain.

We recognise the need for accurate and repeatable methods of measuring pain, but much can be learned about a patient's pain from simple observations. Our assessments are made by looking at the patient's face and watching the way in which he turns over in bed.

We also subscribe to the view that prevention is better than cure, and it is our practice to keep patients free of pain by means of prophylactic analgesics. Some patients are even roused at 5 a.m. for analgesic tablets, but soon go back to sleep, and at 7 a.m., when they waken naturally, they do not have pain, which is a marvellous boost to morale.

Constipation is a problem commonly associated with terminal illness in our experience, and many patients who are admitted with loaded bowels are relieved of rectal pain and dysuria, quite simply by emptying the rectum. The procedure may take several weeks in the frail and elderly, but the effect can be dramatic and has prompted Lammerton to refer to 'resurrection by enemata!'

Pain is not the only symptom with which we are concerned. Dehydration is often found in patients with urinary incontinence who reduce fluid intake in an effort to spare themselves the indignity of their incontinence. In most cases catheterisation and fluid by mouth bring about a remarkable improvement in both general and mental condition, so that return home is possible.

The aims of our treatment are to keep patients alert, to encourage them to enjoy life to the best of their ability, and whenever possible to discharge them to their own homes and families. Time spent at home is increased gradually from an occasional meal at the weekend to, perhaps, a whole weekend and so on until sufficient confidence has been gained for them to remain at home indefinitely. They are visited by a follow-up team.

The work of Saunders (1976, 1973, 1967) and Hinton (1967) has revolutionised our understanding of the needs of the dying, and we encourage both doctors and nurses in training to visit our unit to see our concept of care and the way in which we use drugs.

I am encouraged to find increasing awareness in younger doctors of the need to treat patients rather than symptoms, a sentiment expressed so succinctly by S. Cavenagh in the *British Medical Journal* (1977):

> 'Of course everybody wants better GPs: more knowledge, fuller training programmes, a better balance to keep abreast of modern technological medicine. But finally every patient is going to exhaust, and be exhausted by, the technology and become terminally ill. The qualities then required are not so much techniques but rather the traditional Hippocratic ones of accepting the unacceptable, managing the unmanageable, and bringing hope to the hopeless. At present these seem to be neither deliberately cultivated, nor examined by even the most carefully modified essay question. Yet, before visual aids, peer groups, or age-sex registers were even thought of, those who taught us passed on respect for a few old-fashioned virtues without using the paraphernalia we now seem to find essential.'

To this quotation I would add another for my surgical colleagues, by Henry Troupp (1977):

> 'He', (the surgeon,)'still gets too little advice and help in handling distressed patients. I do not believe that patients' emotional problems should be the exclusive domain of the psychiatrist. Every doctor, except possibly those that have taken permanent refuge in some laboratory, should have a modicum of knowledge in this field. Some are born with the knack; some can never achieve it, but most learn it the hard way, hard for the patients and hard for the doctor.'

The problem of communication between doctor and patient is not new, and the Rock Carling Lecture by Charles Fletcher on this subject, in 1973, in fact stimulated the Nuffield Provincial Trust to fund a study on the problem. 'Medicine seems curiously inept in its communication with its customers', (*British Medical Journal,* 1976).

I believe that adequate communication with patients requires knowledge of their intellectual, cultural, social, emotional and spiritual background and, above all, confidence and complete trust. This takes time to acquire, and is one of the greatest advantages of having patients resident in a special unit with the same staff and a one-to-one-nurse-to-patient ratio. Every day begins with a case conference at which each of our patients is discussed in the minutest detail by medical and nursing staff, and then in the evening I walk round the ward alone and talk to the patients individually. They are surprised that I should know what sort of day they have had, whether the pain has been better or worse, or if they have been sick,and will often talk about problems which may have been of concern for days, weeks or even years.

I no longer think that relief of pain is the most important feature of our work, except in rare cases such as involvement of the brachial or sacral plexus. It is more important to relieve fear and anxiety, and above all to break down tension between patients and their families. Much of my time is spent listening to relatives and patients separately. This is one advantage of admitting patients to a residential unit away from the tensions of the home environment.

As far as reasonably possible, patients should be given freedom and ability to make their own decisions and we encourage them to do what they want. Some patients are terrified of death, their fear based upon a sense of guilt, combined with a childish idea of God as an angry old man wanting to catch us out and to punish us for our misdeeds.

Tranquillizers and the panoply of modern chemotherapy will not help in these circumstances,but reassurance from a trusted physician may succeed, as nothing else will, in convincing the patient that the transition from life to death is not to be feared.

Admission to a special care unit is just one factor in the care of patients with illnesses from which recovery is unlikely. The unit becomes a reference point for the patients and their relatives throughout this worrying and anxious period.

### References

Cavenagh, S., (1977) Personal view, *British Medical Journal*. **I**. 1080.
Fletcher, C.M., (1973) *Communications in Medicine*, London Nuffield Provincial Hospital Trust.
Hinton, J., (1967). *Dying*. London. Pelican.
Leading Article, (1976). Communicating Better. *British Medical Journal*, **I**. 1362.
Saunders, C., (1963) *Proceedings of the Royal Society of Medicine*, 56. No.3 pp. 191–197.
Saunders, C., (1973) *Medical Oncology*, Ed. K.D. Bagshawe, Oxford, Blackwell.
Saunders, C., (1976) Care of the Dying 2nd Ed. *Nursing Times*, **72**, No.26 July 1.
Troupp, H., (1977) Personal view, *British Medical Journal*. **I**. 970.

### Discussion

*Session 6B*

*Dr Robbie.* As radiotherapists are now very much involved in terminal care,may I ask Prof. Joslin for his comments?

*Prof. Joslin.* I do not care for the expression, 'terminal care'; what we are talking about is a form of continuing care and this does not apply merely to cancer patients. One fundamental problem mentioned by Dr Gusterson is that of communication, and this aspect of medicine must be stressed much more in the training of both doctors and nurses. Success in this area leads to greater job satisfaction and in our experience decreases the problems of nurse recruitment.

*Dr West.* I would like to return to the pain problem. It is very important to ensure that the patient has adequate relief and at St Christopher's we do not pursue pain, we anticipate it. I, too, would stress the need for communication,and as I leave a patient's bedside I ask myself, is this person and his family comfortable in body, mind and spirit? If the answer to each question is yes, then one does not have to worry about that patient any more that day.

*Dr Laidlow.* On the question of communication, I find it extraordinary that young, relatively inexperienced housemen are expected to explain the nature of the patient's illness to relatives and to discuss prognosis. I would also make a plea that we discontinue the practice of revealing the diagnosis to the spouse but not to the patient, as this may create family tension, in some cases of long duration.

*Dr Jackson.* When confronted with cancer patients we must not assume that they have not been seen or informed about their illness by some other clinician.

My practice is to stimulate a dialogue in which the patient is encouraged to ask the question to which an honest answer can be given.

*Dr Gusterson.* I would agree that a patient must always be told the truth, but not of necessity the whole truth. We, for example, never use the emotive word 'cancer', which suggests a long, lingering and painful death, but often refer instead to 'some malignancy' a description more readily accepted by the patient.

*Prof. Joslin.* There are a number of emotive key words in this context but I think it is not so much their use but the way in which they are used or qualified which is of importance.

*Prof. Donald.* I have had a cancer successfully excised and as a doctor I can look at the subject objectively, but one thing I do deplore in hospital practice is the conspiracy of silence.

*Dr West.* Probably the most important aspect in 'how much to tell' is as Dr Gusterson mentioned, a complete knowledge of the patient and a complete mutual trusting relationship.

At St Christopher's we answer serious questions truthfully and fully, pointing out, for example, that 'cancer' does not mean prolonged, inevitable, painful death.

I commend the practice of a backward glance when leaving the bedside to see the patient's facial expression, as just occasionally one has to go back and pick up the pieces.

# Session 7 Chairman: J. D. P. Graham

# Buprenorphine

# 19. Pharmacological aspects in man

J. M. ORWIN

## Introduction

A preliminary communication of the respiratory and other effects of buprenorphine compared to morphine,and their reversal with naloxone,was presented at the VI World Congress of Anaesthesiology, Mexico 1976 – section 5,subsection 5,session III. A double-blind comparison of buprenorphine and morphine following intramuscular administration was presented at a Symposium, 'Adjuvant drugs in Anaesthesiology', University of Ghent 1976. The results and tables are reproduced by kind permission of the Editor, Acta Anaesthesiologica Belgica. In the present paper the pharmacological effects of buprenorphine following several routes of administration are described,and comparison with reference compounds discussed. A preliminary communication on the effect of doxapram on buprenorphine-induced respiratory depression is included.

Buprenorphine (N-Cyclopropylmethyl/7 – (1-S-hydroxy, 1, 2, 2, – trimethylpropyl) –6 14 endoethano – 6,7,8 14 tetrahydronororpavine hydrochloride) is a narcotic antagonist analgesic derived from thebaine (Lewis,1974). Studies in rodents and monkeys suggested that buprenorphine would be a long acting efficacious analgesic with a low physical dependence liability (Cowan, Lewis and Macfarlane,1977) and without major effects on the cardiovascular and respiratory systems (Cowan, Doxey and Harry,1977).

Preliminary studies in man using thermal stimulation showed that buprenorphine following intravenous, intramuscular, sublingual and oral administration elevated the experimental pain threshold. Following intramuscular administration,2/$\mu$g/kg buprenorphine gave an equivalent peak effect to 10 mg morphine. The peak effect with buprenorphine persisted up to three hours after administration,whereas following morphine the effect started to decay after one hour.

In a further series of trials the pharmacological profile has been studied following intramuscular, intravenous, sublingual and oral administration of buprenorphine.

## Intramuscular administration

In a pilot study the effects of buprenorphine 0.3 mg and morphine 12.5 mg following intramuscular administration were compared,using a single-blind crossover design in six healthy volunteers monitored for seven hours (Orwin et al,1976a).

Respiratory effects were assessed with the subjects breathing air and by monitoring the displacement of the carbon dioxide response curve using a rebreathing method

141

(Orwin *et al*, 1976a). Effects on heart rate, blood pressure and pupil size were recorded by palpation sphygmomanometry and circular mm scale respectively. Subjective and unwanted effects, as reported by the subjects, were quantified by positioning a movable pointer on a 100 mm scale with 0 = no effect, 100 = effect as bad as it could be. The reverse of the scale was divided into thirds thus, slight (+) moderate (++) and severe (+++) effects. This enabled a standard scoring system to be used and allowed each subject to compare subsequent degrees of effect.

The displacement of carbon dioxide response curve with both drugs was fairly similar though the onset of action of morphine was more rapid than that of buprenorphine. The displacement caused by buprenorphine administration was significantly greater (p$<$0.05) than that caused by morphine at one and a half and four hours after administration, thus identifying a longer peak effect of buprenorphine.

An important clinical feature in this study was that buprenorphine caused significant less of a fall in both systolic and diastolic blood pressure than morphine. Although neit drug caused a significant decrease in heart rate, there was no difference between the treatments and the magnitude of the fall would not be regarded as clinically important. There was a significant reduction in pupil size with both drugs, with no difference between the two treatments. In terms of unwanted effects, moderate degrees of light-headedness, drowsiness and relaxation were observed with both drugs; however with buprenorphine the effects were longer-lasting and persisted into the post-study period.

Following the above pilot study a further double-blind randomised crossover study in six healthy volunteers was carried out. Each volunteer received 5 mg and 10 mg morphine and 0.15 mg, 0.3 mg and 0.6 mg buprenorphine intramuscularly, with at least four days between administrations. The methods have been described in full elsewhere (Orwin, Orwin and Price 1976).

The subjects had a mean age and weight of 27.7 years and 73.8 kg respectively. All data were subjected to an analysis of variance. There was a significant dose response in terms of displacement of the carbon-dioxide response curve between morphine 5 mg and 10 mg at one hour, while buprenorphine reached peak effect at between two and five hours (Table 19.1). Because of the different time effect curves for the two drugs, the relative potency (Fig. 19.1) was determined between

| Drug/Dose | | Time (hr) | | | | | | | |
|---|---|---|---|---|---|---|---|---|---|
| | | ¼ | ½ | 1 | 2 | 3 | 4 | 5 | 6 |
| Morphine | mean | 0.68 | 1.67 | 2.07 | 2.43 | 2.54 | 2.70 | 1.21 | 1.01 |
| 5 mg | SD | 1.74 | 2.13 | 1.44 | 1.40 | 2.17 | 2.23 | 1.20 | 1.07 |
| Morphine | mean | 2.32 | 2.61 | 3.99 | 3.80 | 3.34 | 3.34 | 2.49 | 1.06 |
| 10 mg | SD | 1.56 | 2.63 | 2.82 | 1.64 | 2.06 | 2.32 | 3.13 | 2.86 |
| Buprenorphine | mean | 0.89 | 1.01 | 2.23 | 3.47 | 2.44 | 2.26 | 2.34 | 0.63 |
| 0.15 mg | SD | 1.92 | 1.66 | 2.36 | 3.00 | 2.73 | 2.25 | 2.09 | 1.85 |
| Buprenorphine | mean | 1.63 | 2.91 | 4.25 | 5.31 | 5.80 | 4.99 | 5.78 | 4.76 |
| 0.3 mg | SD | 2.62 | 3.00 | 2.90 | 3.13 | 4.75 | 3.34 | 5.56 | 4.23 |
| Buprenorphine | | 1.58 | 4.15 | 4.95 | 5.30 | 5.81 | 5.91 | 5.89 | 5.34 |
| 0.6 mg | SD | 1.66 | 2.89 | 3.86 | 2.52 | 3.63 | 3.18 | 4.17 | 3.74 |

Mean response ± SD (n = 6) crossover

Table 19.1. Effect of buprenorphine and morphine on displacement of carbon dioxide response curve (mmHg).

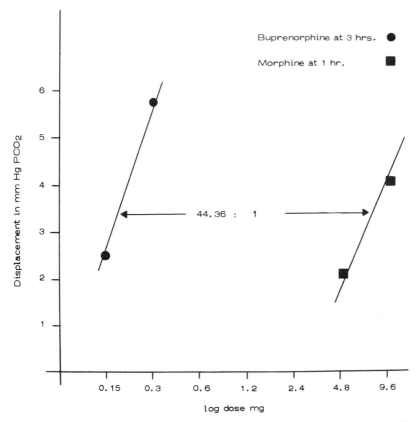

Fig. 19.1. Relative potency of buprenorphine to morphine in terms of respiratory depression at peak.

morphine at one hour and buprenorphine at three hours. This gave a relative potency of 44.36 : 1 with 95% confidence limits of 92.48 and 21.48.

All treatments produced a decrease in the slope of the carbon dioxide response, but the changes were not statistically significant. The end tidal $pCO_2$ with the subjects breathing air reflected the displacement of the carbon dioxide response curve. Only buprenorphine 0.15 mg failed to give a significant increase over the six hours. Over the period one to four hours morphine 10 mg and buprenorphine 0.3 and 0.6 mg gave a similar increase. However, by the fifth and sixth hours the mean for buprenorphine 0.6 mg was significantly greater than morphine 10 mg ($p < 0.001$) and buprenorphine 0.3 mg ($p < 0.01$) (Table 19.2). The falls seen in minute volume only reached significance with buprenorphine 0.3 mg at one, three, four, five and six hours ($p < 0.05$) (Table 19.2). All treatments reduced the tidal volume after 30 minutes but no significant difference between treatments was found. There were only minor falls in respiratory rate. The decrease in respiratory rate seen with the increased dose of buprenorphine was not statistically significant (Table 19.2).

The pulse rate showed a statistically significant fall with each treatment, but no difference between treatments was detected. A reduction in systolic blood pressure was seen with each treatment. For morphine 5 mg the fall was significant only at six

### End Tidal $pCO_2$ (mmHg)

| Drug/dose | | con | ¼ | ½ | 1 | 2 | 3 | 4 | 5 | 6 |
|---|---|---|---|---|---|---|---|---|---|---|
| | | | | | | Time (hr) | | | | |
| Buprenorphine 0.15 mg | | 35.98 | 36.06 | 36.85 | 36.75 | 37.33 | 37.10 | 37.48 | 37.71 | 37.35 |
| | 0.3 mg | 36.50 | 36.59 | 37.28 | 38.58 | 39.30 | 39.88 | 40.43 | 39.28 | 39.00 |
| | 0.6 mg | 36.15 | 37.08 | 38.36 | 39.43 | 40.08 | 38.86 | 40.01 | 40.88 | 40.88 |
| Morphine 5.0 mg | | 34.36 | 34.61 | 35.51 | 36.25 | 36.78 | 35.55 | 37.16 | 36.68 | 36.71 |
| | 10.0 mg | 36.90 | 37.48 | 38.03 | 38.95 | 39.38 | 38.95 | 39.83 | 39.38 | 37.83 |

### Tidal Volume (ml)

| Drug/dose | | con | ¼ | ½ | 1 | 2 | 3 | 4 | 5 | 6 |
|---|---|---|---|---|---|---|---|---|---|---|
| Buprenorphine 0.15 mg | | 619 | 595 | 554 | 596 | 606 | 576 | 538 | 565 | 603 |
| | 0.3 mg | 581 | 605 | 517 | 492 | 543 | 545 | 460 | 488 | 536 |
| | 0.6 mg | 629 | 604 | 543 | 532 | 553 | 567 | 515 | 538 | 521 |
| Morphine 5.0 mg | | 657 | 633 | 579 | 549 | 520 | 646 | 558 | 559 | 576 |
| | 10.0 mg | 574 | 598 | 536 | 519 | 850 | 558 | 506 | 564 | 614 |

### Minute Volume (litre/min)

| Drug/dose | | con | ¼ | ½ | 1 | 2 | 3 | 4 | 5 | 6 |
|---|---|---|---|---|---|---|---|---|---|---|
| Buprenorphine 0.15 mg | | 8.15 | 8.25 | 7.78 | 8.15 | 8.21 | 8.03 | 7.45 | 7.56 | 8.38 |
| | 0.3 mg | 8.35 | 8.05 | 7.90 | 6.71 | 6.78 | 6.71 | 6.20 | 6.28 | 6.60 |
| | 0.6 mg | 8.40 | 7.78 | 6.83 | 6.48 | 6.60 | 7.26 | 6.75 | 6.58 | 6.06 |
| Morphine 5.0 mg | | 9.25 | 8.50 | 8.21 | 7.91 | 7.96 | 8.71 | 7.51 | 7.73 | 7.66 |
| | 10.0 mg | 8.01 | 8.06 | 7.16 | 6.88 | 7.13 | 7.55 | 6.40 | 7.35 | 8.05 |

### Respiratory Rate (per min)

| Drug/dose | | con | ¼ | ½ | 1 | 2 | 3 | 4 | 5 | 6 |
|---|---|---|---|---|---|---|---|---|---|---|
| Buprenorphine 0.15 mg | | 13.1 | 14.0 | 14.1 | 13.5 | 14.1 | 14.1 | 13.8 | 13.8 | 13.8 |
| | 0.3 mg | 14.5 | 14.1 | 15.3 | 13.3 | 12.5 | 12.5 | 13.3 | 12.8 | 12.3 |
| | 0.6 mg | 13.8 | 13.0 | 12.5 | 12.3 | 12.0 | 12.9 | 13.1 | 12.3 | 11.6 |
| Morphine 5.0 mg | | 14.3 | 13.3 | 14.1 | 14.3 | 14.8 | 13.6 | 13.3 | 14.0 | 13.5 |
| | 10.0 mg | 14.0 | 13.6 | 13.5 | 13.1 | 13.0 | 13.3 | 13.0 | 13.1 | 13.3 |

Mean response n = 6

Table 19.2. Effects of buprenorphine and morphine on respiration .

hours ($p < 0.05$); for morphine 10 mg the fall was significant at two hours ($p < 0.05$) and three, four, five and six hours ($p < 0.01$). Buprenorphine 0.15 mg and 0.6 mg produced no significant changes. For buprenorphine 0.3 mg the changes were significant at one, two and four hours ($p < 0.05$).

There were minor falls in diastolic blood pressure with each treatment against time but these did not reach statistical significance. However, the treatment means over the six hour period showed that buprenorphine 0.6 mg gave a significantly greater fall than buprenorphine 0.15 mg ($p < 0.05$). Visual inspection of the e.c.g. revealed no abnormalities. There was a decrease in pupil size with each treatment. This decrease reached statistical significance with buprenorphine 0.3 mg at one to six hours ($p < 0.05$) and with buprenorphine 0.6 mg at one to six hours ($p < 0.05$). The unwanted effects seen with morphine and buprenorphine were qualitatively similar and dose-dependent. Effects seen with morphine were nausea, drowsiness, dizziness and difficulty in concentrating. With buprenorphine lightheadedness, drowsiness and dizziness were the main effects; one subject vomited with each dose of buprenorphine. This appeared worse following 0.3 mg. The effects following buprenorphine were prolonged into the period following the study, and two subjects vomited on becoming ambulant. One subject recorded effects following 0.6 mg lasting up to twenty-four hours.

The difference in mean displacement of the carbon dioxide response curve in these six subjects between 0.3 mg and 0.6 mg buprenorphine was not statistically significant.

To clarify whether this effect was maintained, five of the six subjects received 1.2 mg buprenorphine intramuscularly and the respiratory effects were determined (one subject was excluded because of vomiting on the lower doses). The displacement of the carbon dioxide response curve following this round of medication was increased when compared with the lower doses: this was reflected in the respiratory parameters with the subjects breathing air. The variations in pulse, blood pressure, and pupil size were similar to those observed following 0.6 mg buprenorphine. All subjects developed a degree of sedation and one subject vomited on several occasions. The effects in all subjects were long-lasting, and in three dizziness or lightheadedness persisted for up to twenty-four hours when the subjects became ambulant.

Table 19.3 shows the displacement data for all treatments for the subjects who

| | Time (hr) | | | | | | | |
|---|---|---|---|---|---|---|---|---|
| Dose mg | ¼ | ½ | 1 | 2 | 3 | 4 | 5 | 6 |
| 0.15 | 0.61 | 0.69 | 1.94 | 2.70 | 2.18 | 1.85 | 2.34 | 0.64 |
| 0.3 | 1.50 | 3.41 | 4.30 | 4.07 | 3.82 | 3.82 | 3.61 | 3.17 |
| 0.6 | 1.44 | 3.75 | 4.23 | 4.05 | 4.85 | 5.10 | 4.49 | 4.20 |
| 1.2 | 2.18 | 3.18 | 5.05 | 5.75 | 5.41 | 6.17 | 5.28 | 5.20 |

Mean response n = 5 crossover (subjects 2,3,4,5,6)

Table 19.3. Displacement of carbon dioxide response curve following intramuscular buprenorphine over the dose range 0.15 mg to 1.2 mg.

received the higher dose of buprenorphine. From these figures the mean peak effect between one and six hours was calculated (Table 19.4) and subjected to correlation

| Subject Buprenorphine | 0.15mg | 0.3mg | 0.6mg | 1.2mg |
|---|---|---|---|---|
| 2 | -0.67 | 2.69 | 3.20 | 4.04 |
| 3 | 3.70 | 6.45 | 4.15 | 4.44 |
| 4 | 1.42 | 3.37 | 2.38 | 6.35 |
| 5 | 0.67 | 2.31 | 4.04 | 2.67 |
| 6 | 4.58 | 3.85 | 8.68 | 9.80 |
| Mean | 1.94 | 3.73 | 4.4 | 5.46 |

Table 19.4. Mean peak effects of displacement of carbon dioxide response curve (1–6 hours) subjects 2, 3, 4, 5, 6.

analysis. A statistically significant linear relationship was demonstrated between mean peak effect and dose, ($r = 0.52$ $p < 0.05$) over the dose range 0.15 mg to 1.2 mg buprenorphine (Fig. 19.2).

Thus while the double-blind study suggested that the increase in respiratory depressant effect between 0.3 and 0.6 mg buprenorphine was less than that between 0.15 mg and 0.3 mg, when the data for the subject who did not take part in the further round were removed from the analysis the displacement of the carbon dioxide response curve showed a significantly linear relationship over the dose range 0.15, 0.3, 0.6, and 1.2 mg. The ceiling effect which might have been predicted from the three-point data for the six subjects was not confirmed. The observed linear relationship is in line with that reported by Weldon-Bellville and Green (1965) for pentazocine over the dose range 10 to 40 mg.

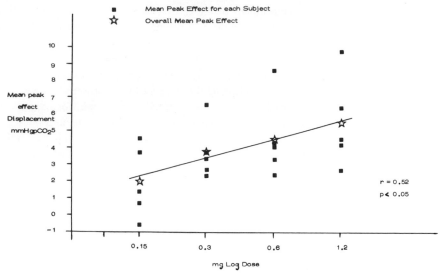

Fig. 19.2. Mean peak effect of displacement of carbon dioxide response curve (1-6 hours) Subjects 2, 3, 4, 5, 6.

## Sublingual administration

The effects of buprenorphine 0.4 mg and 0.8 mg following sublingual administration have been studied in an open, non-crossover trial in two groups of four subjects.

Clinical and respiratory effects were monitored as described earlier. Cardiovascular effects were determined using the non-invasive technique of impedance cardiography (Kubicek *et al* 1974) and systolic time intervals measured and interpreted as described by Aranow (1974) and Spodick and Zambrano (1974). There was a significant displacement of the carbon dioxide response curve following both doses, with a greater displacement following the higher dose, although the difference at the time of peak effect was not statistically significant in these small groups (Table 19.5).

| | Time (hr) | | | | | | |
|---|---|---|---|---|---|---|---|
| | ½ | 1 | 2 | 3 | 4 | 5 | 6 |
| | Buprenorphine 0.4 mg Sublingual | | | | | | |
| Mean | 1.56 | 2.04 | 3.66 | 4.41 | 4.21 | 4.32 | 2.15 |
| SD | 0.74 | 1.95 | 2.14 | 3.36 | 4.30 | 3.00 | 2.63 |
| | Buprenorphine 0.8 mg Sublingual | | | | | | |
| Mean | 1.03 | 2.85 | 4.91 | 5.37 | 5.85 | 3.38 | 4.30 |
| SD | 1.51 | 1.41 | 3.66 | 2.06 | 3.70 | 3.54 | 3.14 |

Mean response ± SD (n=4) non crossover

Table 19.5. Effect of sublingual buprenorphine on displacement of carbon dioxide response curve (mmHg $pCO_2$).

Respiratory parameters with the subjects breathing air tended to reflect this displacement (Fig. 19.3).

The haemodynamic changes seen in both dose groups were relatively small in degree and compensatory mechanisms appeared little affected. The initial effect

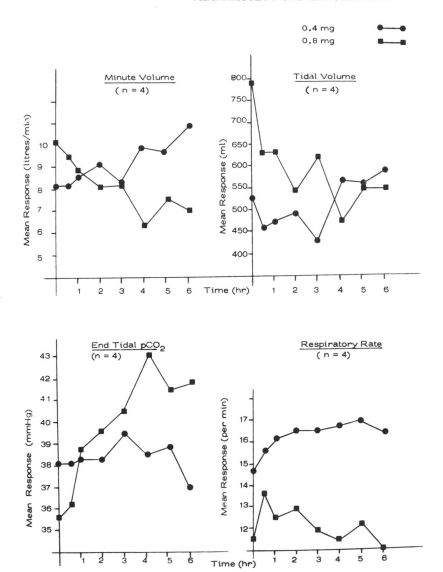

Fig. 19.3. Respiratory effects of sublingual buprenorphine.

appeared to be a lowering of the heart rate. The fall was similar in both dose groups and remained relatively constant for the period of study. The falls in heart rate were associated with increases in stroke volume which appeared immediately in the 0.8 mg group but not until four hours in the 0.4 mg group. This resulted in greater falls in mean cardiac output following 0.4 mg buprenorphine in the first half of the study period (Fig. 19.4).

Peripheral resistance showed minor increases during this period; however, at four hours following 0.4 mg and at three hours following 0.8 mg, falls were observed which were maintained until the end of the period under study. Associated with the

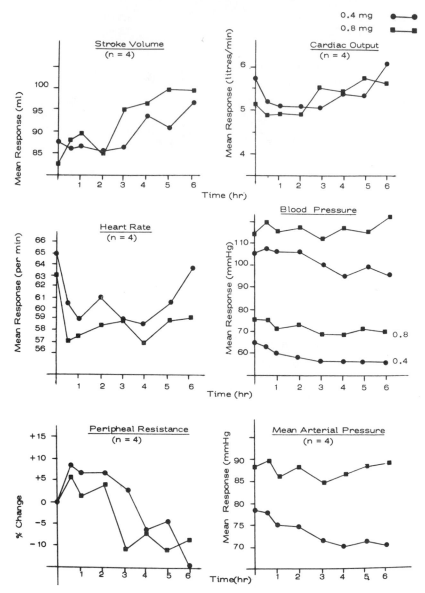

Fig. 19.4. Cardiac effects of sublingual buprenorphine.

falls in peripheral resistance were further increases in stroke volume. These had the effect of increasing the mean cardiac output and of maintaining the mean arterial blood pressure in the 0.8 mg group. In the 0.4 mg group the increases in stroke volume between four and six hours did not fully counteract the falls in peripheral resistance, with decreases in cardiac output still being recorded at four and five hours, however, these decreases were less than those recorded in the first half of the study when compared with control values. Falls in mean arterial blood pressure were found in this group between three and six hours (Fig. 19.4). The systolic time intervals reflected the various haemodynamic changes (Fig. 19.5). Thus the EICT and PEP/LVET fell, and LVET and LVET/EICT increased and appeared associated with the increase in stroke volume at four, five and six hours in the 0.4 mg group*. Similar changes were seen in the 0.8 mg group (i.e. falls in EICT and PEP/LVET and LVET/EICT); however, these were of greater degree and were observed over the whole period of study, reflecting the greater increases seen in stroke volume between thirty minutes to six hours in this group.

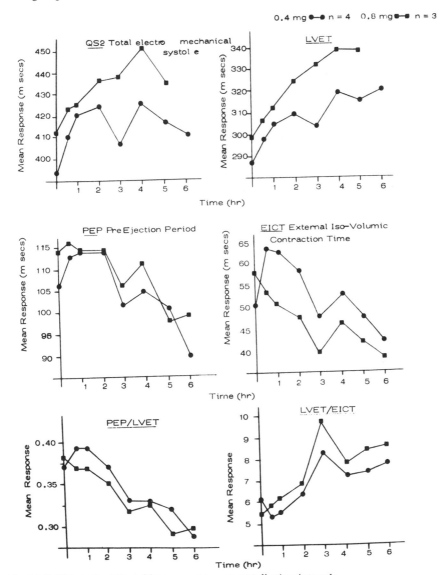

Fig. 19.5. Effect of sublingual buprenorphine on systolic time intervals.

*QS2     Total electro-mechanical systole.
EICT     External iso volumic contraction time.
PEP     Pre-ejection period.
LVET     Left ventricular ejection time.

These characteristic changes in systolic time intervals associated with the rises in stroke volume would indicate that in healthy subjects receiving these doses of buprenorphine there was no significant effect on myocardial contractility. The picture seen in both dose groups in the period three to six hours is consistent with an increase in stroke volume in the presence of a constant inotropic level. (Spodick and Zambrano 1974).

This conclusion is drawn from the observation that there were increases in LVET (in the presence of a relatively stable pulse rate after the initial fall), decreases in PEP, EICT, PEP/LVET and increases in LVET/EICT.

The total electro-mechanical systole (QS2) showed immediate rises in both groups and reflected the changes in heart rate (Spodick and Zambrano, 1974). If the effects had been primarily due to a decrease in after-load at a constant inotropic level, a fall in LVET and QS2 would be expected and similarly, if the effect had been caused by a positive inotropic effect, falls in EICT would have been associated with falls in LVET and QS2 (Spodick and Zambrano, 1974). Thus the increases in QS2 and LVET found with the other effects suggest that the effects observed in the systolic time intervals and ratios are primarily the result of the changes in heart rate and stroke volume, and that these changes are the result of compensatory mechanisms initially brought into play by the decreases in heart rate and in the latter half of the study by falls in peripheral resistance.

Pupillary and subjective effects were similar to those observed following other routes of administration. However, one subject experienced a feeling of detachment with the high dose. The study of haematological and biochemical parameters in blood and urine revealed no changes related to the administration of buprenorphine.

## Sublingual buprenorphine in ambulant subjects

The effects of sublingual buprenorphine have been further studied in ambulant volunteers. In a double-blind randomised crossover study the effects of 0.1 mg, 0.15 mg, 0.2 mg buprenorphine and placebo on heart rate, blood pressure, respiration rate, pupil size and subjective and unwanted effects were compared for a period of seven hours, observations being taken at thirty minutes, one hour and then hourly for seven hours. All subjects (mean age 29.5 years, mean weight 73.2 kg) completed the crossover. The sublingual tablet was well accepted. There were no statistically significant changes in heart rate, blood pressure, respiration rate and pupil size between the four treatments.

However, 0.2 mg buprenorphine produced unwanted effects in significantly ($p < 0.05$) more subjects than all other treatments. Table 19.6 shows the total number of all unwanted effects for the seven hour period. For example, if a subject experienced dizziness over several hours, this would be recorded at each observation time and included in the total. These figures therefore also indicate the difference in the duration of the unwanted effect, those seen with 0.2 mg being of longer duration. Buprenorphine 0.2 mg resulted in significantly more ($p < 0.01$) unwanted effects than placebo, buprenorphine 0.1 mg and 0.15 mg, with no significant difference between placebo, buprenorphine 0.1 mg and 0.15 mg.

The unwanted effects with 0.2 mg became apparent at two hours in eight subjects and at three hours in five subjects. Only one subject was incapacitated on 0.2 mg

Total unwanted effects for each treatment

| | Placebo | Buprenorphine | | |
|---|---|---|---|---|
| | | 0.1 mg | 0.15 mg | 0.2 mg |
| Headache | 1 | 5 | 0 | 6 |
| Lightheaded | 0 | 4 | 3 | 7 |
| Dizzy | 6 | 3 | 4 | 16 |
| Sleepy | 0 | 0 | 0 | 1 |
| Sedated | 0 | 0 | 0 | 10 |
| Nausea | 0 | 0 | 3 | 8 |
| Vomiting | 0 | 0 | 0 | 1 |
| Dry mouth | 0 | 0 | 2 | 2 |
| Sweating | 1 | 0 | 0 | 5 |
| Blurred vision | 0 | 0 | 0 | 3 |
| Happy | 0 | 0 | 0 | 3 |
| Relaxed | 1 | 0 | 2 | 0 |
| Trembling hands | 1 | 0 | 0 | 0 |
| Intoxicated | 0 | 0 | 1 | 0 |
| Inability to concentrate | 0 | 0 | 1 | 0 |
| Queazy | 0 | 0 | 1 | 0 |
| Indifferent | 0 | 0 | 1 | 0 |
| Feeling of well-being | 0 | 2 | 0 | 0 |
| Total | 10 | 14 | 18 | 62 |
| Number of subjects | 4 | 6 | 5 | 14 |

Table 19.6. Total unwanted effects for each treatment.

with dizziness, sweating, nausea and dry mouth. This was partly alleviated by lying down; however, the effects lasted for twelve hours after administration. One subject vomited on one occasion only, three hours after administration of 0.2 mg.

## Oral administration

Preliminary studies in man identified subjective effects following a dose of 1.5 mg/70 kg buprenorphine administered orally. In a further open, single dose trial twelve healthy subjects, divided into three groups of four, were studied using the methods previously described.

The displacement of the carbon dioxide response curve with time in the three dose groups is seen in Figure 19.6. There was a discrete peak effect following 1 mg and 2 mg at two hours and following 4 mg at three hours. However, the effects were still present six hours after administration. The increase in effect with dose was not statistically significant in these small groups.

There was a decrease in the slope of the carbon dioxide response curve (Table 19.7) which was most marked following the higher doses. The respiratory parameters with

152

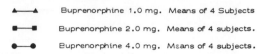

Buprenorphine 1.0 mg.  Means of 4 Subjects

Buprenorphine 2.0 mg.  Means of 4 subjects.

Buprenorphine 4.0 mg.  Means of 4 subjects.

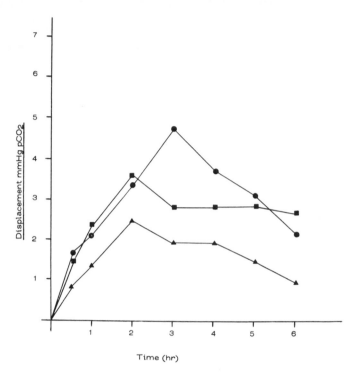

Fig. 19.6. Displacement of respiratory response curve following administration by the oral route (non-crossover).

| Dose (mg) | Time (hr) | | | | | | | |
|---|---|---|---|---|---|---|---|---|
| | control | ½ | 1 | 2 | 3 | 4 | 5 | 6 |
| 1.0 | 2.70 | 2.61 | 3.09 | 2.61 | 2.72 | 2.55 | 3.20 | 3.58 |
| | 0.72 | 0.90 | 1.01 | 0.74 | 1.34 | 0.66 | 1.84 | 1.35 |
| 2.0 | 2.09 | 1.75 | 1.14 | 1.36 | 1.45 | 2.02 | 1.59 | 1.71 |
| | 0.97 | 0.69 | 0.44 | 0.52 | 0.74 | 1.18 | 1.01 | 1.00 |
| 4.0 | 2.35 | 2.29 | 2.56 | 1.97 | 2.09 | 1.91 | 2.63 | 2.29 |
| | 0.52 | 0.74 | 1.28 | 0.47 | 0.63 | 0.28 | 0.52 | 0.69 |

Mean response $\pm$ SD(n = 4)

Table 19.7. Effect of oral buprenorphine on slope of carbon dioxide response curve (Litres/Minute/mmHg).

the subjects breathing air reflected the displacement of the carbon dioxide response curve. Table 19.8 shows these effects.

| Dose (mg) | Control | ½ | 1 | Time (hr) 2 | 3 | 4 | 5 | 6 |
|---|---|---|---|---|---|---|---|---|
| | | | | Minute Volume (litres/minute) | | | | |
| 1.0 | 7.75 1.84 | 7.80 2.36 | 7.97 3.07 | 7.25 1.49 | 7.00 1.46 | 6.75 1.11 | 7.12 1.52 | 7.62 1.34 |
| 2.0 | 8.37 1.68 | 7.75 1.18 | 7.12 1.52 | 6.87 0.89 | 7.12 1.28 | 7.37 1.73 | 7.25 1.18 | 8.50 2.57 |
| 4.0 | 8.70 1.89 | 8.82 2.34 | 8.25 2.25 | 8.27 1.09 | 8.00 1.28 | 7.70 1.05 | 7.67 1.23 | 9.62 0.91 |
| | | | | End Tidal $pCO_2$ (mmHg) | | | | |
| 1.0 | 37.12 4.02 | 37.70 5.00 | 37.17 5.30 | 38.52 4.33 | 38.95 3.97 | 38.70 2.81 | 38.22 4.04 | 37.90 2.47 |
| 2.0 | 36.25 3.53 | 37.57 2.54 | 38.40 3.46 | 38.77 3.70 | 38.40 4.40 | 38.10 3.46 | 37.37 2.80 | 36.92 3.14 |
| 4.0 | 36.77 1.72 | 36.72 1.63 | 37.60 1.73 | 37.45 1.45 | 38.20 1.31 | 38.65 1.24 | 38.40 1.18 | 36.07 1.19 |
| | | | | Respiratory Rate (per minute) | | | | |
| 1.0 | 15.5 4.4 | 15.5 5.2 | 16.0 4.2 | 15.5 3.4 | 15.7 4.6 | 15.5 3.3 | 15.5 4.8 | 16.2 4.7 |
| 2.0 | 14.2 2.6 | 14.2 3.0 | 14.5 5.2 | 13.2 4.8 | 13.7 4.6 | 13.7 5.8 | 14.2 4.7 | 15.2 5.1 |
| 4.0 | 15.0 5.3 | 14.5 5.2 | 15.0 5.1 | 15.5 4.6 | 14.0 4.1 | 13.2 3.9 | 13.7 2.9 | 15.5 3.4 |

Mean response ± SD  (n = 4 )

Table 19.8. Respiratory effects of buprenorphine following oral administration.

Falls in heart rate were seen in each group (Table 19.9). The highest mean fall was found in the 4.0 mg group five hours after administration. Changes in systolic and diastolic blood pressure were quantitatively similar in each group (Table 19.9).

Cardiovascular effects of buprenorphine following oral administration
Heart Rate (per minute)

| Dose (mg) | control | ½ | 1 | Time (hr) 2 | 3 | 4 | 5 | 6 |
|---|---|---|---|---|---|---|---|---|
| 1.0 | 74.00 10.58 | 69.00 8.24 | 70.00 7.65 | 63.00 6.00 | 63.00 10.00 | 63.00 9.45 | 64.00 10.83 | 61.00 11.48 |
| 2.0 | 69.00 12.38 | 62.00 10.06 | 60.00 8.63 | 62.00 10.58 | 56.00 10.32 | 57.00 8.86 | 56.00 8.63 | 59.00 11.01 |
| 4.0 | 74.00 12.43 | 66.00 14.78 | 64.00 15.31 | 62.00 13.26 | 66.00 14.04 | 63.00 16.45 | 57.00 16.12 | 60.00 17.58 |
| | | Blood pressure (mmHg) | | | | | | |
| 1.0 | 110/68 14/5 | 109/66 6/5 | 103/65 10/4 | 98/65 5/6 | 99/64 6/3 | 101/61 10/5 | 100/63 8/6 | 104/65 11/4 |
| 2.0 | 118/66 10/5 | 110/61 14/9 | 108/61 17/9 | 108/63 22/10 | 104/63 19/10 | 105/63 17/10 | 108/61 22/9 | 108/63 17/10 |
| 4.0 | 118/73 13/17 | 113/74 17/18 | 113/71 17/15 | 108/71 15/71 | 103/59 11/14 | 105/68 13/13 | 105/68 13/13 | 108/68 15/12 |

Mean response ± SD   (n = 4 )

Table 19.9. Cardiovascular effects of buprenorphine following oral administration.

Decrease in pupil size (Table 19.10) appeared dose-related and the peak effect following the highest dose was still present six hours after administration. Lightheaded-ness, drowsiness and dry mouth occurred in several subjects during the study period.

| | % decrease | Time of peak effect after administration |
|---|---|---|
| 1.0 mg | 14% | 3 hr |
| 2.0 mg | 23% | 2 – 5 hr |
| 4.0 mg | 27% | 2 – 6 + hr |

Table 19.10 . Mean percentage decrease in pupil diameter (mm) following oral buprenorphine.

However, on becoming ambulant six hours after administration, nausea appeared in several subjects and persisted for 12 + hours; it was however relieved by lying down.

No changes attributable to buprenorphine were found on routine haematological or biochemical examination of blood and urine.

### Reversal of effects of buprenorphine

It is known that larger doses of naloxone are needed to antagonise the agonist actions of narcotic antagonist analgesics than the corresponding actions of morphine. (Kosterlitz, Lord and Watt, 1972). Animal studies confirmed this to be true for buprenorphine, when a ten-fold increase in the dose of diprenorphine was required to effect the same degree of antagonism with the antagonist given thirty minutes after buprenorphine rather than at the same time. In contrast the antagonism of morphine by diprenorphine was little affected by time of injection (Cowan et al, 1977). Antagonism of the effects of buprenorphine by naloxone has been studied in man. (Orwin et al, 1976b).

Five healthy fasting volunteers, (mean age 29 years, mean weight 71.86 kg), were studied.

Respiratory depression was determined by displacement of the carbon dioxide response curve, using a rebreathing method. The effects on other respiratory parameters were determined with the subjects breathing air. Clinical and subjective effects were determined by methods previously described. Following control readings, buprenorphine 0.3 mg was given intravenously. Readings were taken at fifteen minutes and thirty minutes and followed by either naloxone or an equivalent volume of normal saline intravenously. The reversal medications were given in a single-blind randomised manner. Doses of naloxone were: 2.4 mg, 4.0 mg, 8.0 mg, 12.0 mg, 16.0 mg, or an equivalent volume of normal saline. All subjects completed the crossover and thus acted as their own control.

The degree of displacement of the carbon dioxide response curve thirty minutes after buprenorphine was used as the base line. The degree of reversal or further displacement after naloxone or saline in the individual subjects is seen in Table 19.11. This demonstrates the extent of reversal or the degree to which naloxone prevents further respiratory depression occurring. Falls in minute volume and tidal volume were less following naloxone than after saline administration. These two parameters

| Subject | 30 min. | | 60 min. | | 90 min. | |
|---------|----------|--------|----------|--------|----------|--------|
|         | Naloxone | Saline | Naloxone | Saline | Naloxone | Saline |
| 1 | −7% | −111.6% | 37% | −123.8% | 12% | −204.8% |
| 2 | 54% | 14.5% | 43% | −32.4% | 30% | −58.7% |
| 3 | 55% | 18.1% | 84% | −13.2% | 70% | 44.7% |
| 4 | 25% | −3.5% | 30% | −9.2% | 30% | −21.4% |
| 5. | 51% | 4.3% | −30% | 18.8% | 55% | 44.8% |

Negative value indicates further respiratory depression

Table 19.11. Reversal by naloxone or normal saline of respiratory depression following buprenorphine.

also returned to control levels within five to six hours after naloxone whereas in several subjects there was some decrease present at these times following saline reversal.

The end tidal $pCO_2$ rose to a peak at one to two hours following saline reversal, whereas naloxone prevented any further rise and this parameter returned to normal within the period of study (Table 19.12). The number and severity of unwanted effects was decreased following naloxone when compared to saline reversal (Table 19.13) and four of the five subjects reported that they felt 'back to normal' within two to five hours after naloxone whereas the effects persisted for the period of the study following saline. No major changes were observed in the pulse, blood pressure, pupil size or e.c.g. In this study there was evidence of antagonist action persisting for at least five hours. If the mean effect of the three subjects who received the highest doses of naloxone (i.e. 8.0 mg, 12.0 mg and 16.0 mg) is compared to the occasion when they received saline reversal (Fig. 19.7) it will be seen that there was an immediate partial reversal and that the effect of naloxone persisted over the period of study. This was also borne out by these subjects commenting that they felt 'back to normal' during a variable period (two to five hours) following naloxone, after which there was no reappearance of subjective effects of buprenorphine. Evans et al, (1974) found that 0.4 mg/70 kg naloxone would reverse the effects of morphine, but little antagonist effect persisted after forty-five minutes. However, Jasinski, Martin and Sapira (1968) found that 15 mg/70 kg naloxone antagonised the respiratory and other effects of 1 mg/70 kg cyclazocine and that antagonist activity persisted for three to five hours. It would appear that there is an increase in duration of antagonist effect with increase in dose of naloxone. As shown above, the doses of naloxone required to give reversal of the effects of buprenorphine are larger than those required to reverse a pure agonist. Doxapram, a respiratory stimulant, has been shown to decrease the respiratory depression produced by pethidine (Ramamurthy, Steen and Winnie, 1975) and pentazocine (Gasser and Weldon-Bellville, 1975).

Doxapram appears to act by indirect activation of medullary respiratory neurones **via** carotid chemoreceptor activation (Hirsch and Wang, 1974).

| Subject | Buprenorphine followed by naloxone at 30 minutes Time (hr) | | | | | | | | | | | |
|---|---|---|---|---|---|---|---|---|---|---|---|---|
| | 0 | 0.25 | 0.5 | 0.75 | 1 | 1.5 | 2 | 2.5 | 3.5 | 4.5 | 5.5 | 6.5 |
| 1 | 36.5 | 37.8 | 37.8 | 37.8 | 42.8 | 43.5 | 40.6 | 40.6 | 41.3 | 42.8 | 42.8 | 39.2 |
| 2 | 35.3 | 35.3 | 36.3 | 37.8 | 37.5 | 38.9 | 38.2 | 38.9 | 38.2 | 38.2 | 38.2 | 35.3 |
| 3 | 42.2 | 43.7 | 45.8 | 46.5 | 44.4 | 42.2 | 43.7 | 43.7 | 43.7 | 43.7 | 43.7 | - |
| 4 | 33.2 | 28.8 | 38.9 | 38.9 | 40.4 | 38.9 | 35.0 | 38.9 | 34.6 | 30.2 | 31.0 | - |
| 5 | 41.1 | 42.2 | 42.9 | 43.3 | 42.9 | 43.6 | 42.5 | 40.8 | 38.6 | 40.0 | 41.5 | 41.5 |

| Subject | Buprenorphine followed by saline at 30 minutes Time (hr) | | | | | | | | | | | |
|---|---|---|---|---|---|---|---|---|---|---|---|---|
| | 0 | 0.25 | 0.5 | 0.75 | 1 | 1.5 | 2 | 2.5 | 3.5 | 4.5 | 5.5 | 6.5 |
| 1 | 32.9 | 35.0 | 37.9 | 40.7 | 43.6 | 42.2 | 47.9 | 45.0 | 44.3 | 42.2 | 47.9 | 43.0 |
| 2 | 37.2 | 38.6 | 39.4 | 39.4 | 38.6 | 39.4 | 41.5 | 41.5 | 38.6 | 41.5 | 40.8 | 38.6 |
| 3 | 37.8 | 41.4 | 44.9 | 45.6 | 44.9 | 44.9 | 42.8 | 43.7 | 44.2 | 44.2 | 40.6 | 42.8 |
| 4 | 33.9 | 34.6 | 44.0 | 43.2 | 46.9 | 46.9 | 46.8 | 46.8 | 45.4 | 43.9 | 37.5 | 42.5 |
| 5 | 39.9 | 42.05 | 44.95 | 43.50 | 45.68 | 44.95 | 44.93 | 44.23 | 44.95 | 44.23 | 44.23 | 43.5 |

Doses of naloxone:  Subject 1, 2.4 mg; 2, 4.0 mg; 3, 8.0 mg; 4, 12.0 mg

5, 16.0 mg or equivalent volume of normal saline

Table 19.12. Effect on end tidal $pCO_2$ of naloxone or placebo administered 30 minutes after buprenorphine.

| Degree of Effect | Treatment at 0.5 hr. | Unwanted Effects at Various Times | | | | |
|---|---|---|---|---|---|---|
| | | 0 - 0.5 hr. | 0.5 - 1 hr. | 1 - 2 hr. | 2 - 4 hr | 4 - 6 hr |
| Severe | Saline | 3 | 1 | 9 | 2 | Nil |
| | Naloxone | 3 | 1 | Nil | Nil | Nil |
| Moderate | Saline | 8 | 4 | 7 | 7 | 1 |
| | Naloxone | 3 | 4 | 1 | Nil | 1 |
| Mild | Saline | 6 | 4 | 5 | 12 | 13 |
| | Naloxone | 7 | 6 | 11 | 5 | 1 |
| Total Unwanted Effects | Saline | 17 | 9 | 21 | 21 | 14 |
| | Naloxone | 13 | 11 | 12 | 5 | 2 |

Effects include:-  lightheadedness, dry mouth, sedation, sweating, drowsiness, dizziness, relaxed feeling, nausea and vomiting

Table 19.13. Effect of naloxone on incidence and severity of unwanted effects caused by buprenorphine.

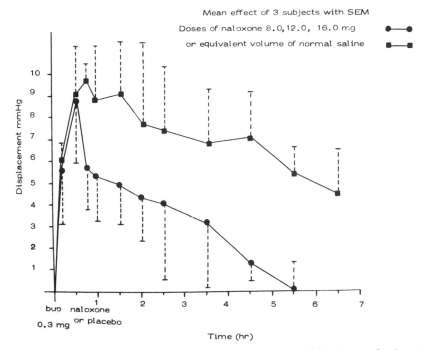

Fig. 19.7. Effect of intravenous naloxone and placebo administered 30 minutes after buprenorphine on displacement of carbon dioxide response curve.

In a blind randomised crossover study in healthy subjects, 0.5 mg/kg and 1.0 mg/kg doxapram compared to placebo produced a dose-dependent respiratory stimulation when administered one hour after buprenorphine (Orwin,1977). Although the profound respiratory stimulant effect was short-lived (approximately ten minutes), comparison with placebo reversal demonstrated that doxapram prevented the peak respiratory depressant effect of buprenorphine, by observation of a decrease in the displacement of the carbon dioxide response curve and the fact that ventilation remained higher after doxapram for several hours. Doxapram infusion produced similar effects (Orwin 1977).

The value of using doxapram to counteract respiratory depression induced by per- and post-operative analgesics has been shown by Arnold *et al*,(1973) and Gupta and Dundee (1974),in that analgesia is maintained,whereas the use of a specific antagonist such as naloxone invariably inhibits analgesia.

## Discussion

The pharmacological profile of buprenorphine has been determined following various routes of administration.

The major pharmacological effects of buprenorphine in man are analgesia, miosis; a variable degree of mental sedation, respiratory depression and a lesser degree of nausea and/or vomiting, which appears exacerbated by movement.

Major psychotomimetic effects, such as have been reported following the use of pentazocine (Jasinski, Martin and Hoeldtke, 1970) and butorphanol (Jasinski D.R., personal communication) have not been observed following administration of buprenorphine to volunteers.

The effects in the dose ranges studied in the series have been dose dependent and of longer duration than reference analgesics. The dose response in terms of respiratory depression was linear over the dose range 0.15 mg to 1.2 mg in volunteers; however, the degree of depression has never been judged to be of clinical significance in patients, even though in one dose-range-finding post-operative study, single doses of buprenorphi up to 7.0 mg (equivalent to approximately 200 mg morphine) were administered intravenously. Lack of clinically significant respiratory effect has subsequently been confirmed by blood gas measurements following administration of 3.0 to 4.0 mg intravenously (Budd, K, personal communication).

It would thus appear that at higher doses there is a marked decrease in the rate of increase of the dose response curve for respiratory depression. A ceiling to the subjective effects at a dose of 1.0 mg buprenorphine following subcutaneous administration has been identified in volunteer studies (Jasinski D.R., personal communication). Effects on the cardiovascular system are of a relatively minor nature; the principal effect being a lowering of heart rate with little effect on contractility. Minor falls in blood pressure have been observed; however, these have been less than the falls observed following equianalgesic doses of morphine. Extensive investigations in a variety of animal species and models have identified a very low physical dependence liability (Cowan et al, 1977). This has been confirmed in human volunteer studies (Jasinski D.R., personal communication) following naloxone challenge and abrupt withdrawal after high dose chronic administration of buprenorphine by the subcutaneo route.

In the search for a potent antagonist analgesic the absence of psychotomimetic effects, the low physical dependence liability, the long duration of analgesic action and the relatively minor effects on the cardiovascular system would represent advantage for buprenorphine over currently available analgesics in this class. While it has not been possible to separate miosis, respiratory depression and the emetic effect from analgesia in this particular compound, these effects have not proved clinically significant in a wide range of doses administered by parenteral, sublingual and oral routes to a wide range of patients with severely painful conditions.

## References

Aranow, W.S. (1974) Post exercise evaluation of ischaemic heart disease by electrocardiography, phonocardiography, apex cardiography and systolic time intervals; in *Non-invasive methods in Cardiology* Ed. S. Zoneraich pp. 244-267. Springfield, Illinois, C.C. Thomas.

Arnold, F.S., Wood, W.B., Morrow, D.H., and Haley, J.V. (1973) Clinical effects of respiratory stimulation with doxapram hydrochloride during neuroleptanalgesia for bronchoscopy. *Anaesthesia and Analgesia Current Researches.* **52,** 643.

Cowan, A., Doxey, J.C., and Harry E.J.R. (1977) The animal pharmacology of buprenorphine, an oripavine analgesic agent. *British Journal of Pharmacology.* In press.

Cowan, A., Lewis, J.W., and Macfarlane, I.R. (1977) Agonist and antagonist properties of buprenorphine. A new narcotic antagonist analgesic. *British Journal of Pharmacology.* In press.

Evans, J.M., Hogg, M.I.J., Lunn, J.N., Rosen, M. (1974) Degree and duration of reversal by naloxone of effects of morphine in conscious subjects. *British Medical Journal* 2, 589.

Gasser, J.C. and Weldon-Bellville, J. (1975) The respiratory effect of doxapram and pentazocine and their interaction. *Anaesthetist,* **24,** 526.

Gupta, P.K. and Dundee, J.W. (1974) The effect of an infusion of doxapram on morphine analgesia. *Anaesthesia,* **29,** 40.

Hennes, H.H. and Osterkamp, E. (1966) Doxapram hydrochlorid (Dopram) und sein Einfluss auf die Ventilationgrossen bei der wachen Versuchsperson. *Anaesthetist,* **15,** 241.

Hirsch, K. and Wang, S.C. (1974) Selective respiratory stimulating action of doxapram compared to pentylene tetrazol. *Journal of Pharmacology and experimental Therapeutics.* **189,** 1.

Jasinski, D.R., Martin, W.R., and Hoeldtke, R.D. (1970). Effects of short and long term administration of pentazocine in man. *Clinical Pharmacology and Therapeutics.* **11,** 385.

Jasinski, D.R., Martin, W.R., and Sapira, J.D. (1968). Antagonism of the subjective, behavioural, papillary and respiratory depressant effects of cyclazocine by naloxone. *Clinical Pharmacology and Therapeutics.* **9,** 215.

Kosterlitz, H.W., Lord J.A.H., and Watt, A.J. (1972). Morphine receptor in the myenteric plexus of the guinea-pig ileum. In *Agonist and Antagonist actions of Narcotic Analgesic Drugs.* Ed. Kosterlitz, H.W., Colloer, H.O.J., Villarreal, J.E. London, Macmillan, pp.45–61.

Kubicek, W.G., Kottke, F.J., Ramos, M.V., Patterson, R.P., Witso, D.A., Labree, J.W., Remole, W., Layman, T.F., Schoening, H., and Garamela, J.J. (1974). The Minnesota impedance cardiograph, theory and applications. *Biomedical Engineering,* **9,** 410.

Lewis, J.W. (1974). Ring C-bridged derivatives of thebaine and oripavine. Narcotic antagonists; in *Advances in Biochemical Psychopharmacology* Eds. Brande, M.C., Harris, L.S., May, E.L., Smith, J.P., Villarreal, J.E., **8,** 123, New York: Raven Press.

Orwin, J.M. (1977) Submitted for publication.

Orwin, J.M., Orwin, J., and Price, M. (1976). A double-blind comparison of buprenorphine and morphine in conscious subjects following administration by the intramuscular route. *Acta Anaesthesiologica Belgica,* **27,** 171.

Orwin, J.M., Robson, P.J., Orwin, J., and Price, M. (1976a). The effects of buprenorphine and morphine on respiration following administration by the intramuscular route in man. Presented at VI World Congress of Anaesthesiology, Mexico, Section 5, sub-section 5, session III, in *Anesthesie et reanimation pratique,* 7, p.157. Ed. Societe d'Anesthesie de Charleroi, Belgique.

Orwin, J.M., Robson, P.J., Orwin, J., and Price, M. (1976b). Antagonist action of naloxone on the acute effects of buprenorphine. Presented at VI World Congress of Anaesthesiology, Mexico, Section 5, sub-section 5, session III, in *Anesthesie et reanimation pratique,* 7, p.189. Ed. Societe d'Anesthesie de Charleroi, Belgique.

Ramamurthy, S., Steen, S.N., and Winnie, A.P. (1975). Doxapram: Antagonism of meperidine-induced respiratory depression. *Anaesthesia and Analgesia Current Research,* **54,** 3, 352.

Spodick, D.H., and Zambrano, S.S. (1974). Investigation of cardiac dynamics by mechanocardiography (systolic time intervals) in *Non-invasive methods in Cardiology,* Ed. S. Zoneraich, pp.296–319, Springfield, Illinois, C.C. Thomas.

Weldon-Bellville, J., and Green, J. (1965). The respiratory and subjective effects of pentazocine. *Clinical Pharmacology and Therapeutics,* **6,** 152.

# 20. A summary of clinical experience in the United Kingdom

A. E. WARD

## Introduction

Strong analgesic drugs are employed widely in the relief of moderate to severe pain. All the drugs available have multiple effects on the patient, most of them mediated through the central nervous system.

Morphine is regarded as the standard of comparison for strong analgesic agents. Seturner isolated morphine as an active ingredient in poppy extract about one hundred years ago (Jaffe and Martin, 1975), and much effort has gone into isolating and synthesising new molecules since that time. The aim has been to retain analgesic potency while reducing or abolishing other, less desirable pharmacological properties.

The profile of a morphine-like analgesic is summarised in Table 20.1. The properties

| i | Analgesia, Sedation, Relief of Anxiety (Euphoria) |
| ii | Sedation, Dizziness, Dysphoria, Nausea, Vomiting, Constipation, Respiratory Depression, Circulatory Depression |
| iii | Tolerance, Dependence |

Table 20.1. The properties of strong analgesics.

shown in section (i) are those which we find desirable and useful; those listed in section (ii) are often termed side effects and may give rise to problems; whereas those in section (iii) are the feared characteristics of the narcotic drugs to which reference has been made in other chapters.

Most of the analgesic compounds developed have been morphine agonists, having the same spectrum of activity as morphine and presumably acting at the same receptors within the central nervous system. They may differ in potency and oral/parenteral efficacy, but all share the side effects listed in Table 20.1.

In the 1950's agents regarded as antagonists to morphine were demonstrated to have analgesic activity. The antagonists were not very potent and had other properties such as hallucinogenic potential, which limited their use. However, interest in antagonist agents has been maintained, because their dependence potential is much less than that of agonist drugs, and other activities like respiratory effects, for example, may not be directly dose related.

160

Buprenorphine is a synthetic molecule demonstrating agonist and antagonist properties and is therefore termed a partial agonist. In clinical and pharmacological studies buprenorphine has been shown to be a potent strong analgesic, and a potent morphine antagonist. The latter property may be employed clinically in the reversal of neurolept analgesia.

It is proposed to outline the profile of buprenorphine in terms of the properties listed in Table 20.1. This is possible because most of the clinical trials have basic features in common. The available information has been coded and with the aid of a computer service, analysed to obtain a general picture of the characteristics of the new drug in clinical use. The data presented are derived from records of more than six hundred parenteral administrations in some 24 studies.

## Study population

The population studied consisted of patients suffering pain resulting from malignant disease or recent surgery, age and weight being fairly evenly distributed throughout the population. In the early studies the dose administered was related to body weight and, females being lighter than males, there was an imbalance in the representation of the sexes at the extremes of the dose range. It was also noted that the patients with cancer had received smaller doses, which probably reflected the low weight of these patients. The presence of a different weight distribution in this sub-group has been confirmed.

The operative procedures were mainly abdominal, but other procedures such as thyroidectomy, mastectomy, thoracotomy, haemorrhoidectomy and limb amputation are included. Patients assessed their pain experience and pain relief according to nominal scales (Table 22.1).

## Pain relief

Pain relief was observed with doses of less than 0.2 mg, but doses of 0.3 mg or more produced better results. (Table 20.2 and 20.3). Differences were observed in the time to onset of relief and the duration of relief, which were related to the route of administration of the drug.

| Buprenorphine (Dose mg) | Cases good/complete relief | Number assessed | % |
|---|---|---|---|
| up to   0.12 | 10 | 16 | 63 |
| 0.13 – 0.22 | 24 | 33 | 72 |
| 0.23 – 0.32 | 54 | 70 | 77 |
| (0.33 – 0.62) | (22) | (37) | (60) |

Table 20.2. Pain relief following intravenous administration of buprenorphine.

| Buprenorphine<br>(Dose mg) | Cases Good/Complete<br>relief | Number<br>assessed | % |
|---|---|---|---|
| up to   0.12 | 62 | 124 | 50 |
| 0.13 − 0.22 | 97 | 138 | 70 |
| 0.23 − 0.32 | 77 | 98 | 79 |
| 0.33 − 0.42 | 24 | 40 | 60 |
| (0.43 − 0.62) | (34) | (42) | (81) |

Table 20.3. Pain relief following intramuscular administration of buprenorphine.

Following intravenous injection the onset of pain relief was rapid, almost 80 per cent of the patients indicating benefit within 15 minutes. The onset of relief was less rapid after intramuscular injection, benefit being reported in the first 30 minutes by 61 cent of patients. By one hour the proportion of patients who reported pain relief had risen to 87 per cent. It appeared that those patients who were to benefit from the analgesic properties of the drug had evidence of this benefit within one hour (Tables 20.4 and 20.5).

| ≪ 15 mins | 16 − 30 mins | 31 − 60 mins | No relief |
|---|---|---|---|
| 91 | 6 | 3 | 15 |
| (79%) | (84%) | (87%) | |

(cumulative percentage figures)

Table 20.4. Onset of pain relief following intravenous administration of buprenorphine.

| up to ½ hour | ½ hour up to 1 hour | 1 hour up to 2 hours | No relief |
|---|---|---|---|
| 283 | 122 | 22 | 40 |
| (61%) | (87%) | (91%) | |

(cumulative percentage figures)

Table 20.5. Onset of pain relief following intramuscular administration of buprenorphine.

There was no apparent relationship between the dose of drug and the time to onset of analgesia. The analgesic effect of a single dose of buprenorphine has been shown to be of long duration. In more than 70 per cent of cases in whom duration was recorded following intravenous injection it equalled or exceeded four hours, and in many cases analgesia persisted for six hours or more (Table 20.6).

| Dose mg | Not recorded | 0 – 1 | 2 – 3 Hours | 4 – 5 | ⟩ 6 | Recorded duration of 4 hours or more |
|---|---|---|---|---|---|---|
| 0.22 | 21 | 3 | 5 | 15 | 10 | 76% |
| 0.23 – 0.32 | 5 | 2 | 10 | 11 | 44 | 82% |
| 0.33 – 0.62 | 17 | 3 | 2 | 7 | 12 | 79% |

Table 20.6. Duration of analgesia following intravenous administration of buprenorphine.

The records of intramuscular injections demonstrated the same prolonged action. The proportion of patients who experienced pain relief of more than four hours' duration approached 82 per cent, and again many patients had benefit for at least six hours (Table 20.7).

| Dose mg | Not recorded | 0 – 1 | 2 – 3 Hours | 4 – 5 | 6 | Recorded duration of 4 hours or more |
|---|---|---|---|---|---|---|
| 0.12 | 10 | 22 | 17 | 30 | 50 | 67% |
| 0.13 – 0.22 | 13 | 14 | 11 | 37 | 72 | 81% |
| 0.23 – 0.32 | 3 | 8 | 9 | 40 | 34 | 81% |
| 0.33 – 0.62 | 5 | 7 | 7 | 26 | 38 | 82% |

Table 20.7. Duration of analgesia following intramuscular administration of buprenorphine.

The results may have been biased against the new analgesic. As observations were usually made at regular intervals for at least six hours, return of pain within this period should have been recorded. It is likely therefore that where a duration of effect was not recorded the analgesia had persisted for longer than six hours.

**Other effects**

The analgesic efficacy of the agent having been demonstrated, its other effects were examined. These may be divided into respiratory effects, cardiovascular effects and side effects observed, or reported by the patient.

The rate of respiration has been measured in most of the studies and in the majority of cases it fell following administration of the analgesic. This change was greater after intravenous than intramuscular injection of the drug, but overall in both instances the observed changes were small, 12 − 15 per cent representing a change in rate of 2 − 4 respirations per minute.

In a very small number of cases the respiratory rate fell to 10 per minute or less. Five of these followed intramuscular injection and 10 cases intravenous injection. Five patients in the latter group were given buprenorphine while under light anaesthesia in a study of respiratory changes.

Pulse rate and systolic and diastolic blood pressures were recorded at set intervals during all the studies. No overall change in pulse rate was demonstrated in association with administration of the analgesic and in individual patients there were no reports of changes of clinical importance.

Again, in individual cases, no changes in blood pressure of clinical importance were observed. All changes seen were within the normal physiological range. Examination of the data from all the intravenous administrations revealed a mean maximum fall in systolic blood pressure of some 10 mm Hg and in diastolic pressure of some 6 mm Hg. Following intramuscular administration the observed mean maximum changes were falls of less than 5 mm Hg for both measurements.

## Side effects

The spectrum of side effects seen with buprenorphine was similar to that seen with other strong analgesic agents, the notable exception having been the absence of dysphoria or psychotomimetic effects. (Tables 20.8 and 20.9). Following intravenous

| Dose mg | Drowsiness or sleeping | Lightheaded or dizzy | Nausea | Vomiting | Sweating | Total Patients |
|---|---|---|---|---|---|---|
| < 0.12 | 11 | 1 | 8 | 2 | 1 | 20 |
| 0.13 – 0.22 | 32 | | 6 | 1 | 2 | 34 |
| 0.23 – 0.32 | 78 | 3 | 23 | 6 | 1 | 74 |
| 0.33 – 0.62 | 41 | 1 | 5 | 10 | | 41 |

Table 20.8. Side effects following intravenous administration of buprenorphine.

administration the most commonly observed side effects were drowsiness and sleep. The incidence of nausea and vomiting, > 20 per cent and > 10 per cent respectively, appeared high and the data were closely examined on these points. It was found that 12 of the 42 patients reported to have experienced nausea were in one study, and that 10 of the 19 reports of vomiting similarly came from one study. These findings may indicate the influence of particular factors in these studies, one of which was the early mobilisation of patients in the study with frequent vomiting. Exclusion of these

| Dose mg | Sleeping or drowsy | Dizzy | Confused | Nausea | Vomiting | Sweating | Total Patients |
|---------|--------------------|-------|----------|--------|----------|----------|----------------|
| ≪  0.12 | 95 | 3 | 1 | 11 | 4 | 4 | 128 |
| 0.13 – 0.22 | 123 | 1 | 1 | 12 | 7 | 8 | 148 |
| 0.23 – 0.32 | 85 | 3 | 1 | 9 | 6 | 6 | 97 |
| 0.33 – 0.42 | 31 | 1 | | 2 | 2 | 2 | 43 |
| 0.43 – 0.62 | 35 | | | 2 | 3 | 1 | 40 |

Table 20.9. Side effects following intramuscular administration of buprenorphine.

cases reduced the incidence of vomiting to 5 per cent. Nausea has been effectively treated in some cases with drugs such as cyclizine.

Nausea and vomiting were less frequent following intramuscular administration, with a recorded incidence of eight per cent and five per cent respectively. It has not been possible to look at tolerance or dependence in the clinical trial situation.

Intramuscular injection of the analgesic was also associated with a high incidence of sedative effects. This did not appear to constitute a problem. Many patients with malignant disease had received drugs to promote sedation and relieve anxiety, and sedation was considered beneficial in the early post-operative period.

## Safety

Doses in excess of 0.6 mg have been used and have not been associated with any different changes in respiratory or cardiovascular function as monitored clinically. The results so far presented have related to doses of $2 - 8\ \mu g/kg$. A number of patients have received $15 - 20\ \mu g/kg$ (unit doses of $1 - 2$ mg) and individual patients have received as much as 7 mg, all without observed ill effect.

## Conclusion

The picture presented is of a potent analgesic, effective in doses of $0.3 - 0.6$ mg by the parenteral route. The analgesic effect is of rapid onset and prolonged duration. Doses in this range are associated with very little disturbance of respiration or cardiovascular function. There is evidence of a number of side effects commonly associated with strong analgesics, but the incidence of effects other than sedation is quite low. It is notable that dysphoria and psychotomimetic effects have not been reported.

From pharmacological and Phase 1 studies it appears that this new drug has a minimal dependence potential, and there is evidence of a wide margin of safety in clinical practice.

### Reference

Jaffe, J.H. and Martin, W.R. (1975) – The Pharmacological Basis of Therapeutics. 5th ed. Goodman, L.S. and Gilman, A. Eds. New York, Macmillan Publishing Co. Inc.

# 21. Clinical trial in post-operative pain

M. M. KAMEL AND I. C. GEDDES

## Introduction

Satisfactory pain relief has always been a difficult problem in clinical practice, and drugs such as opium have been used as analgesics from the earliest period of recorded history. Narcotic analgesics are still indispensable for the treatment of severe pain (Hill and Turner, 1969), and a major objective in analgesic research has been to obtain an agent with the desirable analgesic properties of morphine, but free from its side effects such as addiction and respiratory depression.

Buprenorphine, which was synthesised in 1966, is an N-cyclopropylmethyl oripavine derivative, with a chemical structure closely related to morphine. (See Fig. 11.1).

Lewis (1974) compared its antagonist properties with naloxone and other narcotic antagonists, and in 1976 De Castro and Parmentier summarised the results of animal experiments which showed that it has several interesting properties. It has:

1.  A powerful analgesic action (50 times that of morphine).
2.  A potent morphine – antagonist action (three times that of naloxone).
3.  A weak respiratory depressant activity.
4.  Analgesic potency which does not increase in parallel with respiratory depression, possibly due to its partial agonist action. High doses have been found to stimulate respiration.
5.  A ceiling effect, so that once the intensity of analgesia has reached a certain level higher doses will not increase it. In fact, very high doses reduce the analgesic effect.

Preliminary clinical trials in man have shown that buprenorphine is a safe, potent, long-acting, non-narcotic analgesic useful for post-operative pain relief. (Hovell, 1976).

Morphine has been the standard of comparison in most studies of analgesic action. However, in the present study pethidine was selected, for two reasons:

1.  Pethidine is the standard post-operative analgesic drug given in the ward in which the study was carried out.
2.  A survey on the use of parenteral narcotic analgesics in hospital practice in the West Midlands for the period 1971–1974 has shown that pethidine is the narcotic of first choice in terms of the amount used (Chan, Mitchard and Trueman, 1976).

## Experimental procedure

Sixty consenting adult female patients undergoing gynaecological operations including hysterectomy, tubal surgery and ovarian cystectomy were divided into two equal groups, one group being given buprenorphine 5 $\mu$g/kg and the other group pethidine 1.0 mg/kg. Both drugs were given slowly, but undiluted, by the intravenous route,in the recovery room,and any allergic manifestations or pain due to the injection were recorded 15 and 30 minutes after the injection. All patients were examined at least 24 hours before operation to exclude gross cardiac, respiratory, renal, hepatic or CNS diseases, and they were nursed in the same ward by the same team of nurses.

A standard premedication of 50 mg promethazine was administered orally the night before operation at 10 pm. The anaesthetic technique was also standardised with 2.5 per cent thiopentone as an induction agent, followed by a non-depolarising muscle relaxant (d-tubocurarine or pancuronium). A cuffed oral endotracheal tube was then placed in the trachea under direct vision laryngoscopy, and the cuff inflated. Anaesthesia was maintained by $N_2O$-$O_2$ (70:30) and IPPV with an halothane supplement (less than 0.5 per cent) in some cases. At the end of anaesthesia all patients were reversed by 1.2 mg intravenous atropine and 5.0 mg neostigmine methyl sulphate before extubation. When they were transferred to the recovery room, the patients were awake and co-operative.

## Method of assessment

The following observations were made by the same person. Pain was assessed subjectively (Huskisson, 1974),the degree of severity being scored by the patient as none (0), slight (1), moderate (2), or severe (3). Pulse, blood-pressure and respiratory rate were recorded. Pupil size and reaction to light were recorded. Tidal volume was measured by a Wright's respirometer. A mean of five breaths was recorded. The occurrence of nausea, vomiting, euphoria, dysphoria, anxiety, dizziness, drowsiness, sleep, and sweating were noted and recorded.

There has been a difference of opinion as to whether pain should be measured subjectively, i.e. by the patient, or objectively, i.e. by a trained observer. Parkhouse and Holmes (1963) favoured the use of an objective method, pointing out that some patients are known to exaggerate the severity of their pain. However, we agree with Huskisson (1974) that the severity of pain is known only to the sufferer, and it is difficult to accept that an observer, no matter how experienced, could ever measure another person's pain. We believe that pain is a personal sensation and a psychological experience. If this is accepted, then no observer can play a legitimate part in its direct measurement.

## Results

Table 21.1 gives information on the age and weight distribution of both groups and Table 21.2 shows that they were all well matched for age.

In the ward all observations were carried out hourly by the same person (MMK) for all patients, until a second dose of analgesic was needed or up to a maximum of

168

six hours. All patients were written up for post-operative intramuscular pethidine, but the time of its administration was noted by the ward sister on duty. The nursing staff were informed that the patient had had an analgesic administered before leaving the operating theatre, but did not know which drug was given. An initial attempt to conduct a strict double-blind trial failed because buprenorphine caused a marked miosis within 10 minutes of injection, whereas pethidine did not.

Statistical comparison of the results included:

1. Spearman's rank correlation coefficient between age and duration of analgesia.
2. Student's unpaired t- test for the significance of the difference between two means.
3. Wilcoxon's two – sample test for the differences between mean ranks. (Table 21.3).

| | Buprenorphine | Pethidine GR |
|---|---|---|
| Age (years) | 25 – 67 | 25 – 65 |
| mean | 40.33 | 40.80 |
| S.D. | $\pm4.74$ | $\pm7.74$ |
| Coef. of variation | 11.75% | 16.97% |
| Body weight (Kg) | 50 – 90 | 55 – 85 |
| mean | 64.33 | 63.47 |
| S.D. | $\pm7.49$ | $\pm10.38$ |
| Coef. of variation | 11.61% | 16.37 |
| Number | 30 | 30 |

Age and Weight Distribution of Patients

Table 21.1. Age and weight distribution of patients.

Age distribution of both groups

| | 20 – 29 | 30 – 39 | 40 – 49 | 50 – 59 | 60 – 69 | Total No. |
|---|---|---|---|---|---|---|
| Buprenorphine | 5 | 11 | 7 | 4 | 3 | 30 |
| Pethidine | 3 | 10 | 12 | 3 | 2 | 30 |

$x^2$ = 2.21 (4 d.f.)

P = 0.70 (insignificant)

Table 21.2. Age distribution of both groups.

In the latter test an equivalent formula to the normal approximation, owing to the large numbers and the difference between mean ranks, was approximately corrected for ties.

| Measurement | Time (hours) | Diff. between mean ranks | S.E. of diff. | N.E.D. | 2 - side P |
|---|---|---|---|---|---|
| Respiratory rate | Zero | - 17.30 | 4.47 | 3.87 | 0.00011 *** |
|  | ½ | - 0.77 | 4.47 | 0.17 | 0.86 N.S. |
|  | 1 | - 17.77 | 4.42 | 4.02 | 0.000059 *** |
| Tidal Volume | Zero | + 14.00 | 4.46 | 3.14 | 0.0017 ** |
|  | ½ | + 7.87 | 4.45 | 1.77 | 0.077 N.S. |
|  | 1 | + 10.53 | 4.46 | 2.36 | 0.018 * |
| Pulse Rate | Zero | - 12.07 | 4.48 | 2.69 | 0.0071 ** |
|  | ½ | - 8.87 | 4.45 | 1.99 | 0.046 * |
|  | 1 | - 8.50 | 4.45 | 1.91 | 0.056 N.S. |
| Systolic B.P. | Zero | + 6.50 | 4.41 | 1.47 | 0.14 N.S. |
|  | ½ | + 14.33 | 4.39 | 3.27 | 0.0011 ** |
|  | 1 | - 6.67 | 4.01 | 1.66 | 0.096 N.S. |
| Diastolic B.P. | Zero | - 2.63 | 4.25 | 0.62 | 0.54 N.S. |
|  | ½ | - 0.77 | 4.09 | 0.19 | 0.85 N.S. |
|  | 1 | - 7.53 | 3.70 | 2.04 | 0.042 * |

N.E.D.  =  Normal equivalent deviate

+  =  Buprenorphine > Pethidine

-  =  Buprenorphine < Pethidine

N.S.  =  Not significant

Table 21.3.

Table 21.4 shows the duration of analgesia and dosage for both compounds. Figures 21.1 and 21.2 show the mean pain scores and the mean pain relief respectively. Before drug administration, the mean pain score was slightly higher in the pethidine group, whereas the mean pain relief was slightly higher at 15 minutes, 20 minutes

| | Duration of Analgesia and Dosage | |
|---|---|---|
| | Buprenorphine GR | Pethidine GR |
| Duration of Analgesia | | |
| (hours)  range | 6.0 – 20.0 | 1.5 – 5 |
| mean | 10.57 | 2.63 |
| S.D. | +3.67 | +0.84 |
| S.E.M. | +1.93 | +0.15 |
| Coef. of variation | 34.72% | 31.93% |
| Dose mcg/Kg | 5.0 | 1000 |
| Dose ratio | 1:200 | |
| ratio of mean duration | 4.02:1.00 (10.57) (2.63) | |

Table 21.4. Duration of analgesia and dosage.

and 1 hour in the buprenorphine group. These differences were not statistically signifi-cant (p>0.05). The mean pain relief scores for both groups at 2, 3 and 4 hours were statistically significant (p<0.05). These results are shown in Table 21.5.

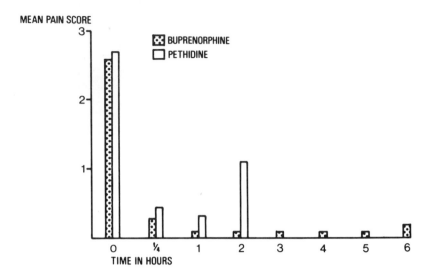

Fig. 21.1. Mean pain relief scores before and after intramuscular injection of buprenorphine and pethidine.

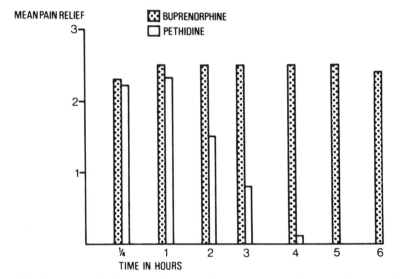

Fig. 21.2. Mean pain relief scores before and after intramuscular injection of buprenorphine and pethidine.

Spearman's rank correlation coefficient between age and duration of analgesia was not significantly different from zero in both groups. Thus, no significant correlation between age and duration of analgesia could be detected in either group. This is shown in Table 21.6.

The changes in respiratory rate and tidal volume were greater in the buprenorphine group 15 minutes after injection, and this was statistically significant ($p < 0.05$). At one hour, however, the difference became insignificant. (Tables 21.7 and 21.8).

| Mean Pain Relief Scores at 1, 2, 3, and 4 hours | | | |
| --- | --- | --- | --- |
| 1 h | 2 h | 3 h | 4 h |
| Buprenorphine  2.50 | 2.50 | 2.50 | 2.50 |
| Pethidine  2.35 | 1.51 | 0.80 | 0.05 |
| Ratio | (1.67/1) | (3.13/1) | (50/1) |

Table 21.5. Mean relief scores at 1, 2, 3, and 4 hours.

| Spearman's Rank Correlation Coefficient (R s) between Age and Duration of Analgesia | | |
| --- | --- | --- |
| Rs | t (29 d.f.) | P |
| Buprenorphine  − 0.096 | 0.51 | 0.61 |
| Pethidine  + 0.132 | 0.71 | 0.49 |

d.f.  =  degrees of freedom

Table 21.6. Spearman's rank correlation coefficient (Rs) between age and duration of analgesia.

| Changes in the Respiratory Rate | | |
| --- | --- | --- |
| | Number of Patients | |
| Increase | Decrease | No change |
| **Respiratory Rate** | | |
| At ¼ hour | | |
| buprenorphine  9  range: 1 – 12/min  mean: 4.33 | 19  range: 1 – 8/min  mean: 3.84 | 2 |
| pethidine  one  20 – 25/min | 29  range: 2 – 9/min  mean: 5.69 | zero |
| At 1 hour | | |
| buprenorphine  3  range: 3 – 6/min  mean: 4.33 | 24  range: 1 – 14/min  mean: 5.54 | 3 |
| pethidine  zero | 29  range: 2 – 8/min  mean: 5.17 | one |

Table 21.7. Changes in the respiratory rate.

| Tidal Volume | Changes in Tidal Volume Number of Patients | | |
|---|---|---|---|
| | Increase | Decrease | No change |
| **At ¼ hour** | | | |
| buprenorphine | 15 range: 20 – 280 ml mean: 110 – 71 ml | 14 range: 30 160 mean: 68 ml | one |
| pethidine | 17 range: 50 – 150 ml mean: 60 ml | 13 range: 20 – 150 ml mean: 59.17 ml | zero |
| **At 1 hour** | | | |
| buprenorphine | 26 range: 20 – 400 ml mean: 150.38 ml | one 50 ml | 3 |
| pethidine | 27 range: 30 – 300 ml mean: 126.67 ml | zero | 3 |

Table 21.8. Changes in tidal volume.

The pulse rate was diminished in both groups, but to a lesser degree in the buprenorphine group. The difference was insignificant at 15 minutes but significant ($p < 0.05$) at one hour. (Table 21.9 and Fig. 21.3).

| | Changes in Pulse Rate Number of Patients | | |
|---|---|---|---|
| | Increase | Decrease | No change |
| **At ¼ hour** | | | |
| buprenorphine | 4 range: 4 – 5/min mean: 4.25 | 23 range: 4 – 30/min mean: 15.09 | 3 |
| pethidine | One 5/min | 27 range: 5 – 30/min mean: 18.81 | 2 |
| **At 1 hour** | | | |
| buprenorphine | 9 range: 4 – 10/min mean: 5.44 | 18 range: 5 – 30/min mean: 16.96 | 3 |
| pethidine | 5 range: 5 – 10/min mean: 7.6 | 23 range: 5 –30/min mean: 16.96 | 2 |

Table 21.9. Changes in pulse rate.

The drop in systolic blood pressure was significantly ($p < 0.05$) less with buprenorphine 15 minutes after injection, whereas the difference between both groups was insignificant at 1 hour. On the other hand, the drop in diastolic blood pressure became significantly greater in the buprenorphine group only at 1 hour. (Table 21.10 and Fig. 21.3).

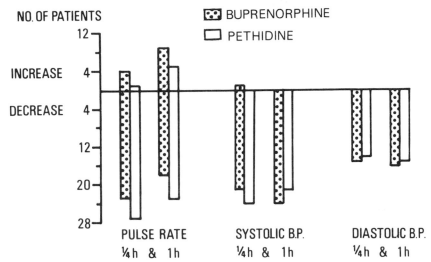

Fig. 21.3. Number of patients with changes in pulse rate, diastolic and systolic blood pressure after intramuscular injections of buprenorphine and pethidine.

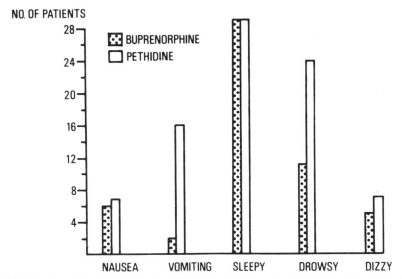

Fig. 21.4 Number of patients with side effects after intramuscular injections of buprenorphine and pethidine.

Figure 21.4 shows that the incidences of vomiting, drowsiness and dizziness were lower with buprenorphine, whereas those of nausea and sleepiness were almost equal in both groups. No allergic side effects, euphoria, dysphoria, pain on injection, nor any serious side effects were recorded in either group.

| Changes in Systolic and Diastolic B.P. | | | |
|---|---|---|---|
| | | Number of Patients | |
| | Increase | Decrease | No change |
| **Systolic B.P.** | | | |
| At ¼ hour buprenorphine | One | 21 range: 10 – 30 mm Hg mean: 15.71 | 8 |
|       pethidine | Zero | 24 range: 10 – 40 mm Hg mean: 17.71 | 6 |
| At 1 hour buprenorphine | Zero | 24 range: 10 – 60 mm Hg mean: 23.33 | 6 |
|       pethidine | Zero | 21 range: 10 – 30 mm Hg mean: 12.86 | 9 |
| **Diastolic B.P.** | | | |
| At ¼ hour buprenorphine | Zero | 15 range: 10 – 30 mm Hg mean: 10.33 | 15 |
|       pethidine | Zero | 14 range: 10 – 20 mm Hg mean: 12.50 | 16 |
| At 1 hour buprenorphine | Zero | 16 range: 05 – 30 mm Hg mean: 13.13 | 14 |
|       pethidine | Zero | 15 range: 5 – 20 mm Hg mean: 9.67 | 15 |

Table 21.10. Changes in systolic and diastolic B.P.

## Discussion

Post-operative pain relief is of great concern to anaesthetists and particularly to those interested in recovery rooms and post-operative intensive care units. A large number of analgesic agents are now available for the management of pain, but no drug has supplanted morphine. Much unnecessary suffering takes place because doctors and nurses are concerned that repeated administration of narcotic drugs to control pain can lead to addiction. Thus, the introduction of a potent non-addictive analgesic drug with no serious side effects would be a great advantage.

Rolly and Versichelen (1976) have shown that buprenorphine, given by intramuscular injection 4 $\mu$g/kg for post-operative pain, produced good analgesia in 73 per cent of their patients and fair analgesia in another 23 per cent. They concluded that a long duration of action and a low incidence of side effects were the main clinical features of this drug. In their study, the mean duration of analgesia obtained was six hours $\pm$ 22 minutes. However, buprenorphine was not administered until there was a demand for pain relief, 90 $\pm$ 5.9 minutes after the end of anaesthesia.

In our study, buprenorphine (5 $\mu$g/kg) was administered intravenously in the immediate post-anaesthetic period before the patient returned to the ward. The analgesia obtained was very satisfactory in all cases with a mean duration of 10.5 hours $\pm$ 3.67. This long duration of pain relief, together with a low incidence of side effects, led to its rapid acceptance by the nursing staff, who are usually resistant to any change in technique.

## References

Chan, K., Mitchard, M. and Trueman, G. (1976). The use of narcotic analgesics in hospital practice. *Journal of clinical Pharmacology*, **1**, 153.

De Castro, J. and Parmentier, P. (1976). Buprenorphine in analgesic anaesthesia. Presented at: VI World Congress of Anaesthesiology, Mexico, Section 5, sub-section 5. pp. 3–13. Ed. Société d'Anesthésie de Charleroi, Belgium.

Hill, R.C. and Turner, P. (1969). Importance of initial pain in post-operative assessment of analgesic drugs. *Journal of Clinical Pharmacology*, **9**, 321–327.

Hovell, B.C. (1976). Buprenorphine (RX 6029–M). Clinical trial in post-operative pain by the intramuscular route. *VI World Congress of Anaesthesiology*, Mexico, 387, 18, Excerpta Medica, International Congress Series.

Huskisson, E.C. (1974). Measurement of Pain. *Lancet*, **2**, 1127–1131.

Lewis, J.W. (1974). Ring C-bridged derivatives of thebaine and oripavine. Narcotic antagonists; in *Advances in Biochemical Psycho-pharmacology*, M.C. Braude, L.S. Harris, E.L. May, J.P. Smith and J.E. Villarreal, Eds. New York, Raven Press, 8, p.123.

Parkhouse, J. Holmes, C.M. (1963). Assessing post-operative pain relief. *Proceedings of the Royal Society of Medicine*, **56**, 579.

Rolly, G. Versichelen, L. (1976). Experience with a new analgesic drug. Buprenorphine. *VI World Congress of Anaesthesiology*, Mexico, 387, 19. Excerpta Medica, International Congress series.

# 22. Comparative studies

B. C. HOVELL

This paper summarises my experiences with buprenorphine given intramuscularly and describes two clinical trials.

## Comparison of buprenorphine, pentazocine and pethidine

The first study was designed to assess the analgesic activity of a number of different single intramuscular doses of buprenorphine (in a double-blind non-crossover trial) using pethidine and pentazocine as reference analgesics. The condition studied was that of early post-operative pain after major or intermediate surgery.

Pre- and per-operative analgesics were avoided, in consenting patients who were observed immediately after operation and, on the first complaint of pain, were given an intramuscular injection of either $2 \mu$g/kg buprenorphine, $4 \mu$g/kg buprenorphine, 1 mg/kg pethidine or 0.6 mg/kg pentazocine. In a supplementary trial with the same protocol $8 \mu$g/kg buprenorphine was given.

Patients were observed at fixed times during the next four hours by trained nurse observers, who observed and recorded pain intensity and the degree of relief by means of similar widely used nominal scales (Table 22.1). Both subjective and objective side effects were noted.

| Type of Pain | Numerical Score | Relief | Score |
|---|---|---|---|
| None | 0 | None | 0 |
| Slight | 1 | Slight | 1 |
| Moderate | 2 | Moderate | 2 |
| Severe | 3 | Good | 3 |
| | | Complete | 4 |

Table 22.1. Nominal scales for measuring pain intensity and pain relief.

*Results*

Pain intensity differences from pre-injection levels were found for each patient for varying periods of time up to four hours both at rest and on limited movement. Mean pain intensity differences for each treatment group were then plotted against time.

It can be seen quite clearly that with the patient at rest the greatest relief of pain was obtained from buprenorphine at 8 μg/kg (Fig. 22.1) followed by buprenorphine 4 μg/kg, buprenorphine 2 μg/kg, pentazocine 0.6 mg/kg and pethidine at 1 mg/kg in descending order of effect. The rate of onset and the peak activity of the drugs were similar. The pain intensity differences were summed and a one-way analysis of variance was then used to test for significant differences between the mean and sum of pain

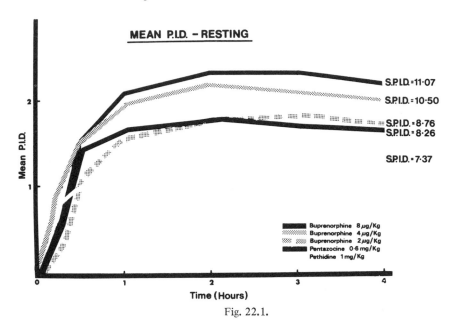

Fig. 22.1.

intensity difference (S.P.I.D.) for the groups of patients having each treatment. The S.P.I.D. scores for buprenorphine 4 μg/kg and buprenorphine 8 μg/kg are both significantly higher than that for buprenorphine 2 μg/kg ($p < 0.05$). Both buprenorphine 4 μg/kg and buprenorphine 8 μg/kg had significantly higher S.P.I.D. than pethidine, ($p < 0.01$) but only the highest dose of buprenorphine resulted in a S.P.I.D. score significantly greater than pentazocine ($p < 0.05$).

The results were also graphed for pain intensity differences on movement and coughing, with similar results (Fig. 22.2). Table 22.2 demonstrates a relationship between dose and pain relief (at rest) for buprenorphine, both buprenorphine 4 μg/kg and buprenorphine 8 μg/kg giving significantly higher S.P.I.D. scores than buprenorphine 2 μg/kg. The only significant difference in the between-drug comparisons is that between the S.P.I.D. scores for buprenorphine 8 μg/kg and pethidine 1 mg/kg ($p < 0.05$).

*Side effects*

The commonest side effect was sedation. Buprenorphine at 8 μg/kg appeared to be

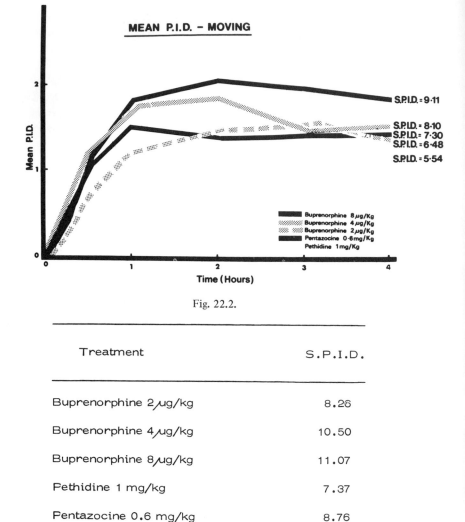

Fig. 22.2.

| Treatment | S.P.I.D. |
|---|---|
| Buprenorphine 2 µg/kg | 8.26 |
| Buprenorphine 4 µg/kg | 10.50 |
| Buprenorphine 8 µg/kg | 11.07 |
| Pethidine 1 mg/kg | 7.37 |
| Pentazocine 0.6 mg/kg | 8.76 |

Table 22.2. Calculated S.P.I.D. scores for the five treatments.

more soporofic than the other treatments. Nausea and vomiting were very uncommon in this series with no detectable difference between the treatment groups. No other significant side effects were noted.

Blood-pressure, pulse rate and respiration rate were monitored, but changes were difficult to interpret in the relatively unstable early post-operative period, and no direct effects could be associated with any one drug, other than bradypnoea on two occasions, following the higher dose of buprenorphine.

## Comparison of buprenorphine and morphine

In the second trial using a very similar protocol a fixed dose of 0.3 mg buprenorphine was compared with 10 mg morphine. Both analgesics were given by intramuscular injection.

*Results*
50 patients were treated and both groups were well matched for age, sex and weight. Pain intensity difference, etc. were plotted against time as in the previous trial, though for the longer period of six hours. There was a statistically significant difference ($p < 0.01$) in the pain intensity difference scores (Figs. 22.3 and 22.4) for six hours after the injection, a dose of 0.3 mg buprenorphine providing better pain relief than 10 mg morphine.

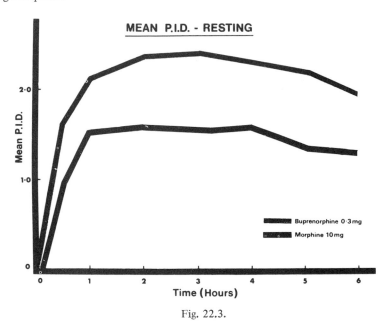

Fig. 22.3.

*Side effects*
The side effects in this second trial were similar to those in the first trial.

## Conclusion

These two trials have shown that buprenorphine is a clinically useful strong analgesic in the post-operative patient. It promises to be long-acting, though in this work measurements were only continued for a maximum of six hours. In these trials the only side effects of note were sedation, from which patients were normally easily aroused. Over the whole of my experiences with the drug, marked slowing of the respiratory rate occurred in approximately 3 per cent of cases, including those where buprenorphine had been given by the intramuscular and sublingual routes, the picture

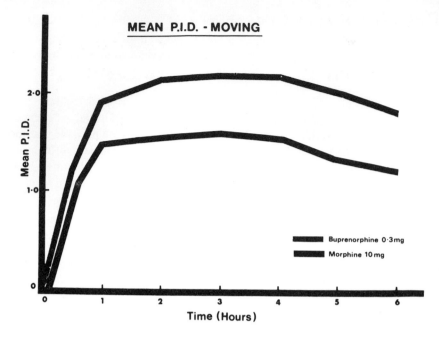

Fig. 22.4

being reminiscent of that seen with phenoperidine. Clinically this has not proved to be a problem.

0.3 mg of buprenorphine intramuscularly appears to be a satisfactory dose in the post-operative situation.

# 23. A study comparing intravenous buprenorphine, morphine and pentazocine in post-operative pain relief

M. E. DODSON, A. HUSSAIN AND H. MATHESON

## Methods

### Subjects

68 patients undergoing hysterectomy were studied. They were fit, free from serious disease, and not on any regular analgesic medication. A brief explanation was given at the pre-operative visit so that they would not be worried by repeated visits from an observer post-operatively.

The pre-medication consisted of promethazine 25 mg intramuscularly one hour before operation, and some patients were also given 10 mg of diazepam orally three hours pre-operatively. A standard anaesthetic of thiopentone, pancuronium, nitrous oxide and halothane was used, and the muscle relaxant was reversed at the end of the procedure using 2.5 mg of neostigmine and 1 mg of atropine.

### Administration of analgesic

The nurses in the recovery room decided when the patient required analgesia. The drugs were presented in randomly numbered identical ampoules. 1 ml of the ampoule was diluted with 9 ml of water, so that each ml of diluted solution contained the dose per 10 kg body weight, i.e. 20 $\mu$g of buprenorphine, 1.5 mg morphine, or 3 mg of pentazocine. The diluted solution was given over five minutes until either the patient's pain was relieved, or a maximum dose of 2 $\mu$g (or later 4 $\mu$g) per kilogram of buprenorphine, 150 $\mu$g per kilogram of morphine, or 300 $\mu$g per kilogram of pentazocin had been given. The dose of buprenorphine was increased to 4 $\mu$g per kilogram after 22 patients had entered into the study, as other work had suggested that this might be a more appropriate dose.

### Observations

Observations on the first 49 patients commenced 10 minutes after giving the drug, and continued every hour for five hours, or until another dose of analgesic was required. At these times, measurements were made of pulse, blood-pressure and respiratory rate. Pain and sedation were assessed and scored. The pain scale was from 0 to 3, 0 being no pain or the patient deeply asleep, 1 mild pain, 2 moderate pain and 3 severe pain. No assessment of pain relief was made, as at this early stage after operation the patients often could not remember what the pain had been like previously. Sedation was similarly scored on a 0 to 3 scale. No sedation (0 score) was given to the patient who was awake when the observer arrived. 1 was the score

182

for the patient who opened her eyes as the observer approached the bed, 2 if she woke only when pulse or blood pressure was taken, and 3 if she did not wake during the time of observations. No attempt was made to wake the patients to answer questions if sedation of grade 3 was present. All the patients except those heavily sedated were questioned about side effects such as nausea, vomiting, dizziness and dreams, and the nurses were also questioned.

24 hours after the operation, the patients were again interviewed. They were questioned about how they felt, how much pain they had had, what sort of night they had had and any side effects. A record was made of the time of all analgesics given during the 24 hours from the end of their operation. The nurses were also questioned, as patients often did not remember episodes of nausea or vomiting.

The subsequent 19 patients were studied in less detail, and only buprenorphine and morphine were compared. Routine ward observations, at hourly intervals, of pulse and blood-pressure were made and also the incidence of nausea and vomiting. The duration of the initial dose of analgesic and the subsequent requirements for analgesia during the first 24 hours were also noted.

### Results

The drug dosage and number of patients are shown in Table 23.1 for each group, and Table 23.2 shows the ages and weights of the patients.

| CODE | PLANNED DOSE / kg | ACTUAL DOSE RANGE / kg | PATIENTS | |
|---|---|---|---|---|
| B2 | BUPRENORPHINE 2 µg | 1.9–2.1 µg | 8 | (8) |
| B4 | BUPRENORPHINE 4 µg | 3.0–4.1 µg | 19 | (9) |
| M | MORPHINE 0.15 mg | 0.1–0.15 mg | 25 | (16) |
| P | PENTAZOCINE 0.3 mg | 0.13–0.31 mg | 16 | (16) |

Table 23.1. Dose and number of patients treated in each group.

| | B2 | B4 | M | P |
|---|---|---|---|---|
| MEAN WEIGHT ( kg ) | 56.5 | 61.4 | 64.5 | 59.3 |
| RANGE | 45–69 | 46–76 | 44–92 | 45–90 |
| MEAN AGE ( yrs ) | 42 | 41.5 | 39 | 36.4 |
| RANGE | 34–49 | 23–55 | 26–61 | 26–52 |

Table 23.2: Distribution of weight and age in the treatment groups.

*Pain scores*
The mean pain score was calculated for the pre-drug observations, and each post-operative observation. The results are shown in Figure 23.1. Each point does not

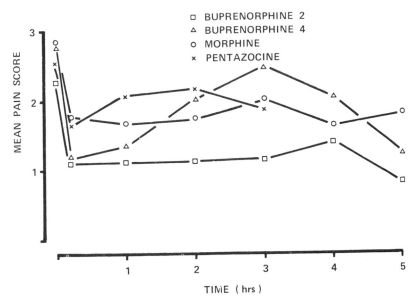

Fig. 23.1. Mean pain scores before and after injection of strong analgesic.

represent a large number of patients, and in some of the later points a mean of only five scores is given. It is obvious, therefore, that no statistically significant differences can be demonstrated for these drugs, but each provided reasonably effective analgesia.

*Sedation scores*
The mean sedation scores are shown in Figure 23.2. Again, the paucity of numbers means that no significant differences are seen, but it looks as though buprenorphine 4 $\mu$g/kg may be more sedative than the other drug regimens.

*Duration of analgesia*
Duration of analgesia was calculated as the time from administration of the test drug to the time when the patient described her pain as severe, had very little sedation, and was considered to need a further dose of analgesic. The decision was made by the observers if within five hours of giving the drug, or by the nursing staff if the duration of analgesia lasted more than five hours. The results are shown in Table 23.3, and it can be seen that both doses of buprenorphine produced a longer mean duration of analgesia than either morphine or pentazocine. The very wide range of duration of analgesia for all these drugs can also be seen. Table 23.4 shows the significant differences between the drugs. Pentazocine is significantly shorter than both doses of buprenorphine, and buprenorphine 4 $\mu$g/kg produced significantly longer duration of analgesia than morphine.

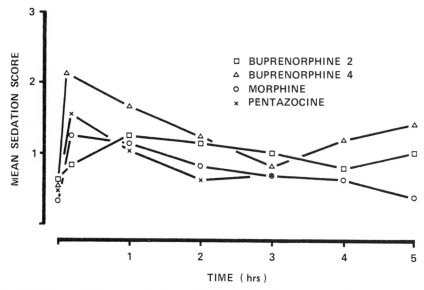

Fig. 23.2. Mean sedation scores before and after injection of strong analgesic.

| Group | Duration of Analgesia (hours) | | |
|---|---|---|---|
| | Mean | S D | Range |
| B2 | 6.43 | 3.47 | 2.25 – 12 |
| B4 | 7.39 | 4.23 | 2.25 – 18 |
| M | 4.88 | 2.96 | 1.25 – 15 |
| P | 3.23 | 1.79 | 1.5 – 7 |

Table 23.3. Mean duration of analgesia after injection of strong analgesic.

| | Significance |
|---|---|
| B2 & P | $p < 0.01$ |
| B4 & M | $0.05 > p > 0.02$ |
| B4 & P | $p < 0.01$ |

Table 23.4. Significance of differences in duration of analgesia between the groups.

*Side effects*
The incidence of the principal side effects is shown in Table 23.5. The results for both

| Group | Incidence of Side-Effects (per cent) | | |
|---|---|---|---|
| | Dizziness | Nausea | Vomiting |
| B2 & B4 | 41 | 65 | 19 |
| M | 55 | 56 | 8 |
| P | 39 | 56 | 6 |

Table 23.5. Incidence of side-effects (per cent).

doses of buprenorphine have been combined, as the numbers in which side effects were recorded were small. None of these differences were significant. It is perhaps worth noting that the nausea, so frequently present, was usually a very transient side effect. Only in two patients, who had the larger dose of buprenorphine, was it severe and persistent. This does suggest that possibly nausea and vomiting are slightly more common with buprenorphine, but many more patients would have to be studied to demonstrate significance.

Dreams were only mentioned by one patient in the whole series, although this was specifically asked about, particularly in view of the occasional hallucinatory effects of pentazocine. This suggests that pentazocine may be free from these side effects when it is given in the early post-operative period, when other anaesthetic drugs are still having an effect.

Two patients had complete amnesia for the whole of the day of the operation after the larger dose of buprenorphine.

The 24-hour observations did not demonstrate any longer-term benefits or disadvantages which could be attributed to the longer action of buprenorphine. The number of doses of intramuscular papaveretum required during the first 24 hours was similar for all three drugs, though there was a trend towards a slightly larger number of doses being required after pentazocine.

*Respiratory effects*
The respiratory rate dropped sharply within 10 minutes of intravenous administration of all three test drugs. Thereafter, the rate remained remarkably stable, and there were no differences between the drugs in the degree of slowing of the respiratory rate.

*Cardiovascular effects*
No significant changes in blood-pressure occurred. The only differences between the drugs were observed in the 10-minute pulse measurements. After morphine and pentazocine, the pulse rate dropped compared with the pre-drug level, but it increased after buprenorphine. This difference almost reached the significance level of $p = 0.05$. A decrease in the pulse rate at 10 minutes would be expected, due to the persistence

of the effects of the anticholinesterase given at the end of the operation, and there is a possibility that buprenorphine may reverse or prevent this effect. Later pulse-rate changes were very similar for all three drugs.

## Discussion

The measurement of pain and its relief presents considerable problems, especially when the patient is drowsy and still under the influence of anaesthetic drugs. A simple method of patient assessment of degree of pain was therefore chosen in this study. Observer assessment of pain was also made, and frequently differed from patient assessment. However, the value of an analgesic agent lies in whether the patient receiving it finds it effective, and therefore only patient assessment of pain was used in the analysis. It is hardly surprising that no differences in degree of analgesia between the drugs were observed using this crude method on a small number of patients, but all drugs were in fact shown to be effective analgesics.

The intravenous route of administration was chosen to avoid problems due to variations in absorption after intramuscular administration. Thus a clear starting point for assessing the duration of analgesia was obtained.

One of the most surprising observations was the very marked variation in the duration of analgesia, some patients getting virtually no pain relief with any of the intravenous test drugs. All these patients responded satisfactorily to intramuscular papaveretum. Despite this variability, a significantly greater duration of analgesia was observed after the larger dose of intravenous buprenorphine.

Side effects were similar with all the drugs, with perhaps a trend towards greater sedation and slightly more nausea and vomiting with buprenorphine.

## Conclusion

Buprenorphine, in the dose of 4 $\mu$g per kilogram intravenously, gave a mean duration of analgesia post-operatively of 7.39 hours, a significantly longer duration than that given by morphine intravenously. The incidence of side effects was similar in type and degree to morphine. This suggests that buprenorphine presents an advance in post-operative analgesia in that fewer injections may be needed to provide satisfactory pain relief.

# 24. Early experience of a six-hourly regimen in post-operative pain

E. REES-JONES

## Introduction

This is a preliminary report of an open study in which buprenorphine is being used as the sole analgesic in a selected group of post-operative patients.

## Methods

Patients who have undergone abdominal, gynaecological or orthopaedic procedures are eligible for the study, but those who have been taking analgesics, hypnotics or anti-depressants pre-operatively are excluded. Day cases and patients with significant respiratory depression are also excluded.

Standard premedication and anaesthetic procedures are followed. Patients are premedicated with Ativan 2.5 mg and Droperidol 10 mg an hour and a half before operation. Anaesthesia is induced and maintained with Althesin, Valium, oxygen and Fluothane. Alloferin is given as a muscle relaxant.

No analgesic is given post-operatively until the patient complains of pain. Buprenorphine 0.3 mg is then given by intramuscular injection and repeated at six-hourly intervals.

Observations including patients' assessment of pain on a nominal scale (Table 22.1), respiration rate, pulse rate and blood pressure are recorded immediately before the first injection and at intervals of three hours thereafter. Side effects reported by the patients in response to open questions, or observed by the nursing and medical staff, are recorded.

## Results

There has been adequate pain relief after the first injection in 26 of the 27 patients studied so far, and this has continued throughout the observation period.

The one patient in whom pain was not relieved by the first injection had good relief after a second dose of buprenorphine.

No clinically significant changes in respiratory rate have been observed, the lowest rate recorded being 16/minute. A respiratory rate of 26/minute noted in one patient during the first six-hour observation period subsequently decreased spontaneously.

It is likely that pulse rates which vary from 72/minute to 120/minute reflect the interplay of complex factors in the early post-operative period, rather than a direct effect of buprenorphine.

Records show a trend for both systolic and diastolic blood-pressure to fall by small amounts after injection. In only one patient, in whom a blood-pressure of 80/50 mm Hg was recorded five hours after the first analgesic injection, was the fall in blood-pressure clinically significant. This patient had a pre-operative blood-pressure of 110/80 mm Hg and an immediately post-operative blood-pressure, before analgesic injection, of 90/60 mm Hg. It is of note that three hours after the second injection of buprenorphine the pressure rose to 120/60 mm Hg.

*Side effects*

Sedation was the most common side effect. The majority of patients appeared to be asleep, but could be aroused without difficulty and were easy to communicate with, once awake. One patient complained of nausea after cholecystectomy and one, who was elderly and confused before operation, continued to be very restless and confused during the study period.

**Conclusions**

Good analgesia has been achieved and maintained in post-operative patients by six-hourly intramuscular injection of 0.3 mg buprenorphine. In comparison with other commonly used strong analgesics there appears to be a qualitative difference in pain relief which is difficult to define. Staff in the unit have suggested that it resembles epidural analgesia.

Sedation, although common, has not been a problem and may account for small falls in blood-pressure which have been observed.

There is no evidence so far in this study of cumulative effects of buprenorphine on respiration, pulse rate or blood-pressure, and there has been no apparent change in the nature or severity of side effects.

**Discussion**

*Session 7*

*Prof. Graham.* Dr Kamel, you showed a score for sleepiness and drowsiness; could you explain the difference?

*Dr Kamel.* After buprenorphine, patients were sleepy, some actually asleep but easily aroused, whereas with pethidine they were drowsy even when wakened.

*Prof. Campbell.* Several speakers commented that there were no psychotomimetic effects after buprenorphine or control drugs. How were the patients questioned, what observations were made and what was understood by psychotomimetic?

*Dr Ward.* In some of the studies patients were questioned directly but on the whole open questions were asked. Apart from being questioned about pain, patients were asked how they felt, to elicit any subjective effects.

In addition, the observers are trained to identify if a patient is disorientated or reacting abnormally, and this was recorded. Classical psychological scoring techniques have not been used in these studies.

*Dr Rees-Jones.* Psychotomimetic effects of other compounds have been identified with this method, and gross effects with buprenorphine would certainly have been noted

*Dr Raftery.* May I ask how the sublingual buprenorphine was formulated and how long did it take to achieve effective levels?

*Dr Orwin.* Sublingual buprenorphine was administered as a small slightly convex round tablet approximately 6 mm in diameter. The subjects were instructed to hold it under the tongue until it dissolved. In our studies the mean time for tablets to dissolve was 4 − 5 minutes, and there was no irritation of the sublingual space. In a subsequent study it took 14 minutes for the tablet to dissolve in one subject and on that occasion he complained of an unpleasant taste persisting for 20 − 30 minutes. With regard to effect we found approximately 30 per cent of peak effect at 30 minutes when studying the displacement of the $CO_2$ response curve.

*Dr Masson.* In clinical practice I have found that it takes about one hour before full effect is achieved.

*Dr Robbie.* I have a wide experience with sublingual buprenorphine at doses of 0.15 mg − 0.8 mg. Results have shown that 0.4 mg is comparable to the analgesics dihydrocodeine and pentazocine, but quicker acting and longer lasting.

One outstanding feature is the ability to produce adequate pain relief without inflicting constipation on the patient. We have found the sublingual preparation peculiarly advantageous in treatment of patients with head and neck cancer, who may find it difficult to swallow tablets and in whom it is beneficial not to have to resort to repeated injections.

*Dr Tate.* In a pilot study we found slight sedation and dizziness within an hour. Nausea and vomiting appeared only after five or six hours, but was short-lived. Can this be explained?

*Dr Orwin.* In our volunteer studies we have found nausea and vomiting at earlier times in subjects who are obviously sensitive to this type of molecule, but certainly in subjects who only became ambulant after a six to seven hour experimental period these effects have been precipitated by movement.

*Dr Budd.* Titrating buprenorphine intravenously to give complete pain relief, we have worked up to a dose of 3 to 4 mg. Following this we see none of the side effects mentioned, but achieve prolonged analgesia, and in fact some of our patients are ambulant three to four hours after cessation of surgery. Although Dr Orwin has identified respiratory depression in volunteers, we have found no evidence of this either clinically or by determination of blood gases, up to six hours after administration of 3 to 4 mg buprenorphine. This has even been the case after doses of up to 7 mg and one patient with terminal malignancy, whose pain was unresponsive to other agents, including large doses of diamorphine, was given 28 mg buprenorphine intravenously with no effect on her respiration or level of consciousness. There was a beneficial analgesic effect.

*Dr Lewis.* Studies of blood gases in conscious rats have shown a polyphasic dose response curve different to morphine or pentazocine. However, at the higher doses, while the blood gases appeared relatively normal, other toxic effects were apparent.

*Dr Geddes.* Is there a method for measuring buprenorphine blood levels?

*Dr Orwin.* A radio-immunoassay is being developed for buprenorphine. In a single volunteer crossover study immuno-reactive buprenorphine was identified following intravenous and sublingual administration. The effect on displacement of the $CO_2$ response curve did correlate with blood level but with a time lag, as would be expected, as this effect is mediated by brain levels.

# Index